Clinical Skills for OSCEs

Life is short, the art long, opportunity fleeting,

experiment treacherous, judgement difficult.

Hippocrates (c. 460–370 BC). Aphorisms, Aph. 1.

Clinical Skills for OSCEs

Third Edition

Edited by
Neel Burton
Teaching Associate, Green College,
University of Oxford

Contributing authors
Neel Burton
Thomas Stockmann
Kuldip Birdi
Akbar de' Medici
Nicholas Stacey

Scion

Third edition © Neel Burton, 2009

ISBN 978 1 904842 59 0

First edition published in 2003 by BIOS Scientific Publishers (ISBN 1 85996 340 4)

Second edition published in 2006 by Informa Healthcare (ISBN 978 1 84184 616 3)

A CIP catalogue record for this book is available from the British Library.

Scion Publishing Limited
Bloxham Mill, Barford Road, Bloxham, Oxfordshire OX15 4FF
www.scionpublishing.com

Important Note from the Publisher

Typeset by Phoenix Photosetting, Chatham, Kent, UK
Printed by Gutenberg Press, Malta

Contents

I.   GENERAL SKILLS

II.   CARDIOVASCULAR AND RESPIRATORY MEDICINE

III.   GI MEDICINE AND UROLOGY

IV. NEUROLOGY

V. PSYCHIATRY

VI. ENT, OPHTHALMOLOGY, AND DERMATOLOGY

VII. PAEDIATRICS AND GERIATRICS

VIII. OBSTETRICS, GYNAECOLOGY, AND SEXUAL HEALTH

IX. ORTHOPAEDICS AND RHEUMATOLOGY

X. EMERGENCY MEDICINE AND ANAESTHESIOLOGY

XI. DATA INTERPRETATION

XII. PRESCRIBING AND ADMINISTRATIVE SKILLS

XIII. COMMUNICATION SKILLS

This third edition of CSFO is largely the product of the many comments and suggestions received from students over the years, principally from the United Kingdom but also from as far afield as Australia, Japan, and the USA. For this third edition, many changes have been made and the contents have been re-organised and expanded to create a section on data interpretation. Although background information has been added in certain areas, this has not jeopardised the clarity and concision of earlier editions. Topics that have benefitted from expansion include some of those most likely to grey your hair, such as ordering and interpreting blood tests and prescribing drugs on hospital drug charts.

This third edition stands out from previous editions not just for its content, but also for its larger size and more colourful appearance. The introduction of full colour, proudly promulgated by the surf shop cover design, serves to enliven the text and support the introduction of colour coding and colour photographs. This should make key information even easier to find, learn, and recall.

I hope that CSFO 3e contributes to making you a better doctor, and that you invest the time and efforts that it saves you on your outside interests. In the long run, being a good doctor is about being a real person, and only you can teach yourself that.

Neel Burton
Oxford, July 2008

Post-scriptum: Comments about this book and suggestions for improving it can be made to neel.burton@green.ox.ac.uk.

Clinical skills exams, such as Objective Structured Clinical Examinations (OSCEs), are a daunting but essential component of medical undergraduate education.

To prepare for these exams, our generation of medical students had to pull together vast amounts of information from maladapted resources. This tedious and time-consuming process can now be avoided, as all this information has been compiled into this one, handy book.

Indeed, this book covers all the clinical skills that are likely to be tested during the clinical years of a medical course. Although it aims to be comprehensive and detailed, its primary purpose is to be easy to read and to the point. *Clinical Skills for OSCEs* does not attempt to teach its reader medicine or surgery, but rather gathers and organises a large amount of information and presents it in a structured and memorable fashion.

We hope you find *Clinical Skills for OSCEs* useful both for your revision and for the consolidation of skills learnt at the patient's bedside.

Neel L Burton
Akbar H de' Medici
Nicholas C Stacey
London, August 2002

- **Don't panic.** Be philosophical about your exams. Put them into perspective. And remember that as long as you do your bit, you are statistically very unlikely to fail. Book a holiday to a sunny Greek island starting on the day after your exams to help focus your attention.

- **Read the instructions carefully and stick to them.** Sometimes it's just possible to have revised so much that you no longer 'see' the instructions and just fire out the bullet points like an automatic gun. If you forget the instructions or the actor looks at you like Caliban in the mirror, ask to read the instructions again. A related point is this: pay careful attention to the facial expression of the actor or examiner. Just as an ECG monitor provides live indirect feedback on the heart's performance, so the actor or examiner's facial expression provides live indirect feedback on your performance, the only difference being – I'm sure you'll agree – that facial expressions are far easier to read than ECG monitors.

- **Quickly survey the cubicle for the equipment and materials provided.** You can be sure that items such as hand disinfectant, a tendon hammer, a sharps bin, or a box of tissues are not just random objects that the examiner later plans to take home.

- **First impressions count.** You never get a second chance to make a good first impression. As much of your future career depends on it, make sure that you get off to an early start. And who knows? You might even fool yourself.

- **Prefer breadth to depth.** Marks are normally distributed across a number of relevant domains, such that you score more marks for touching upon a large number of domains than for exploring any one domain in great depth. Do this only if you have time, if it seems particularly relevant, or if you are specifically asked. Perhaps ironically, touching upon a large number of domains makes you look more focussed, and therefore safer and more competent.

- **Don't let the examiners put you off or hold you back.** If they are being difficult, that's their problem, not yours. Or at least, it's everyone's problem, not yours. And remember that all that is gold does not glitter; a difficult examiner may be a hidden gem.

- **Be genuine.** This is easier said than done, but then even actors are people. By convincing yourself that the OSCE stations are real situations, you are much more likely to score highly with the actors, if only by 'remembering' to treat them like real patients. This may hand you a merit over a pass and, in borderline situations, a pass over a fail. Although they never seem to think so, students usually fail OSCEs through poor communications skills and lack of empathy, not through lack of studying and poor memory.

- **Enjoy yourself.** After all, you did choose to be there, and you probably chose wisely. If you do badly in one station, try to put it behind you. It's not for nothing that psychiatrists refer to 'repression' as a 'defence mechanism', and a selectively bad memory will put you at great ease with you conscience.

- **Keep to time but do not appear rushed.** If you don't finish by the first bell, simply tell the examiner what else needs to be said or done, or tell him indirectly by telling the patient, e.g. "Can we make another appointment to give us more time to go through your treatment options?" Then summarise and conclude. Students often think that tight protocols impress examiners, but looking slick and natural and handing over some control to the patient is often far more impressive. And probably easier.

- **Be nice to the patient.** Have I already said this? Introduce yourself, shake hands, smile, even joke if it seems appropriate – it makes life easier for everyone, including yourself. Remember to explain everything to the patient as you go along, to ask him about pain before you touch him, and to thank him on the second bell. The patient holds the key to the station, and he may hand it to you on a silver platter if you seem deserving enough. That having been said, if you reach the end of the station and feel that something is amiss, there's no harm in gently reminding him, e.g. "Is there anything else that you feel is important but that we haven't had time to talk about?" Nudge-nudge.

- **Take a step back to jump further.** Last minute cramming is not going to magically turn you into a good doctor, so spend the day before the exam relaxing and sharpening your mind. Go to the country, play some sports, rent out a DVD. And make sure that you are tired enough to fall asleep by a reasonable hour.

- **Finally, remember to practise, practise, and practise.** Look at the bright side of things: at least you're not going to be alone, and there are going to be plenty of opportunities for good conversations, good laughs, and good meals. You might even make lifelong friends in the process. And then go off to that Greek island.

Hand washing

Hands must be washed before every episode of care that involves direct contact with a patient's skin, their food, invasive devices, or dressings, and after any activity or contact that potentially contaminates the hands.

The procedure

- Turn on the hot and cold taps with your elbows and wait until the water is warm.
- Thoroughly wet your hands.
- Apply liquid soap or disinfectant from the dispenser. Liquid soap is used in most hospital situations. Disinfectants include aqueous chlorhexidine ('Hibiscrub') and povidone iodine ('Betadine'). Alcohol hand rubs offer a practical alternative to soaps and disinfectants.
- Wash your hands using the Ayliffe hand washing technique (see *Figure 1* overleaf):
  ① palm to palm
  ② right palm over left dorsum and left palm over right dorsum
  ③ palm to palm with fingers interlaced
  ④ back of fingers to opposing palms with fingers interlocked
  ⑤ rotational rubbing of right thumb clasped in left palm and left thumb clasped in right palm
  ⑥ rotational rubbing, backwards and forwards, with clasped fingers of right hand in left palm and clasped fingers of left hand in right palm.
- Rinse your hands thoroughly.
- Turn the taps off with your elbows.
- Dry your hands with a paper towel and discard it in the foot-operated bin, remembering to use the pedal rather than your clean hands!
- Consider applying an emollient.

Station 1 Hand washing

Figure 1. Ayliffe hand washing technique:
  1.1 Palm to palm
  1.2 Right palm over left dorsum and left palm over right dorsum
  1.3 Palm to palm fingers interlaced
  1.4 Backs of fingers to opposing palms with fingers interlocked
  1.5 Rotational rubbing of right thumb clasped in left palm and vice versa
  1.6 Rotational rubbing, backwards and forwards with clasped fingers of right hand in left palm and vice versa

Scrubbing up for theatre

Before handwashing

State that you would:

- Change into scrubs.
- Put on clogs or plastic overshoes.
- Don a theatre cap, tucking all your hair underneath it.
- Remove all items of jewellery, including your watch.
- Enter the scrubbing room.
- Put on a face mask, and ensure that it covers both your nose and mouth.
- Open a sterile gown pack *without touching the gown*.
- Lay out a pair of sterile gloves *without touching the gloves*.

Handwashing

- Open a brush packet containing a nail brush and nail pick.
- Open the taps.

 From here on, keep your hands above your elbows at all times.

The social wash

- Wash your hands with soap, lathering up your arms to 2 cm above the elbows.

The second wash

- Use the nail pick from the brush packet to clean under your fingernails.
- Dispense soap on to the sponge side of the brush and use the sponge to scrub from the fingertips to 2 cm above the elbows (30 seconds per arm).

 Dispense soap using your elbow or a foot pedal, not your hands.

- To rinse, start from your hands and move down to your elbows so that the rinse water does not re-contaminate your hands.

The third wash

- Using the brush side of the brush, scrub your fingernails (30 seconds per arm).
- Using the sponge side of the brush, scrub:
  - each finger and interdigital space in turn (30 seconds per arm)
  - the palm and back of your hands (30 seconds per arm)
  - your forearm, moving up circumferentially to 2 cm above the elbows (30 seconds per arm)

 Remember to keep the brush well-soaped at all times.

- To rinse, start from your hands and move down to your elbows.
- Turn the taps off with your elbows.

After handwashing

- Use the towels in the gown pack to dry your arms from the fingertips down.
- Pick up the gown from the inside, ensuring that it does not touch anything.
- Put your arms through the sleeves, but do not put your hands through the cuffs.
- Put on the gloves without touching the outside of the gloves. Practise this – it's not easy!
- Ask an assistant to tie up the gown for you.

 After scrubbing up, keep your hands in front of your chest and do not touch any non-sterile areas, including your mask and hat.

Venepuncture/phlebotomy

Specifications: The station consists of an anatomical arm and all the equipment that might be required. Assume that the anatomical arm is a patient and take blood from it.

Before starting

- Introduce yourself to the patient.
- Explain the procedure and ask for his consent to carry it out.
- Ask him which arm he prefers to have blood taken from.
- Ensure that he is comfortable.

The equipment

In a tray, gather:

- A pair of non-sterile gloves.
- A tourniquet.
- Alcohol wipes.
- A 12G needle and needle-holder.
- The bottles appropriate for the tests that you are sending for (these vary from hospital to hospital, but are generally yellow for biochemistry, purple for haematology, pink for group and save and crossmatch, blue for clotting, grey for glucose, and black for ESR).
- Cotton wool.

 Make sure you have a sharps bin close at hand. The key to passing this station is to be seen to be safe.

The procedure

- Select a vein: the bigger and straighter the better.
- Apply the tourniquet, and re-check the vein.
- Put on gloves.
- Clean the venepuncture site using the alcohol wipes. Explain that the alcohol wipes may feel a little cold.
- Attach the needle to the needle holder.
- Tell the patient to expect a 'sharp scratch'.
- Retract the skin to stabilise the vein and insert the needle into the vein.
- Keeping the needle still, place a bottle on the needle-holder and let it fill.
- Once all the necessary bottles are filled, release the tourniquet.
- Remove the needle from the vein and apply pressure on the puncture site.
- Dispose of the needle in the sharps bin.
- Remove gloves.

After the procedure

- Ensure that the patient is comfortable.
- Thank the patient.
- Label the bottles (at least: patient's name, date of birth, and hospital number; date and time of blood collection).
- Fill in the form (at least: patient's name, date of birth, and hospital number; date of blood collection; tests required).

Examiner's questions

If the veins are not apparent

- Lower the arm over the bedside.
- Ask the patient to exercise his arm by repeatedly clenching his fist.
- Gently tap the venepuncture site with two fingers.
- Apply a warm compress to the venepuncture site.
- Do not cause undue pain to the patient by trying over and over again – call a more experienced colleague instead.
- Use femoral stab as a last resort.

In the event of a needlestick injury

- Encourage bleeding, wash with soap and running water.
- Immediately report the injury to the local Public Health Consultant.
- If there is a significant risk of HIV, post-exposure prophylaxis should be started as soon as possible.
- Fill out an incident form.

For more information on the management of needlestick injury, refer to local or national protocols.

Cannulation and setting up a drip

Specifications: The station is likely to require you either to cannulate an anatomical arm and to put up a drip, or simply to cannulate the anatomical arm. This chapter covers both scenarios.

Before starting

- Introduce yourself to the patient.
- Explain the procedure and ask for his consent to carry it out.
- Gather equipment in a tray.

 It is important to read the instructions for the station carefully. If, for example, the instructions specify that the patient is under general anaesthesia, you are probably not going to gain any marks for explaining the procedure.

Cannulation only

The equipment

In a tray, gather:
 	
  • A pair of non-sterile gloves.
  • A tourniquet.
  • Alcohol swabs.
  • An IV cannula of appropriate size (*Table 1*). Size is primarily determined by the viscosity of the fluid to be infused and the required rate of infusion.
  • A pre-filled 5 ml syringe containing saline flush.
  • An adhesive plaster.
  • A sharps box.

The procedure

- Find a suitable vein. Try to avoid the dorsum of the hand and the antecubital fossa.
- Apply the tourniquet to the arm and re-verify the vein.
- Put on the gloves.
- Clean the skin with an alcohol swab and let it dry.
- Remove the cannula from its packaging and remove its cap.
- Tell the patient to expect a 'sharp scratch'.
- Anchor the vein by stretching the skin and insert the cannula at an angle of approximately 30 degrees.
- Once a flashback is seen, advance the cannula and needle by about 2 mm.
- Pull back slightly on the needle and advance the cannula into the vein.
- Release the tourniquet.
- Press on the vein over the tip of the cannula, remove the needle completely, and cap the cannula.
- Immediately put the needle into the sharps box.
- Apply the adhesive plaster to fix the cannula.
- Flush the cannula.

General skills

Table 1. IV cannulae		
Colour	**Size**	**Water flow (ml/min)***
Blue	22G	33
Pink	20G	54
Green	18G	80
White	17G	125
Grey	16G	180
Orange	14G	270

* Approximate values. According to Poiseuille's Law, the velocity of a Newtonian fluid through a cylindrical tube is directly proportional to the fourth power of its radius.

After the procedure

- Discard any rubbish.
- Ensure that the patient is comfortable.
- Thank the patient.

Cannulation and setting up a drip

The equipment

In a tray, gather:

- A pair of gloves.
- A tourniquet.
- Alcohol swabs.
- An IV cannula of appropriate size.
- An adhesive plaster.
- A sharps box.
- An appropriate fluid bag.
- A giving set.

The procedure

- Check the fluid prescription chart (if appropriate).
- Check the fluid in the bag and its expiry date.
- Remove the fluid bag from its packaging and hang it up on a drip stand.
- Remove the giving set from its packaging.
- Remove the protective covering from the exit port at the bottom end of the fluid bag.
- Remove the plastic cover from the large, pointed end of the giving set.
- Drive the large, pointed end of the giving set into the exit port at the bottom end of the fluid bag.
- Remove the protective cap from the other end of the giving set.
- Close the roller in the middle of the giving set's tubing.
- Squeeze and release the collecting chamber of the giving set until it is about half full.
- Open the roller and run fluid through the giving set to expel any air/bubbles.
- Close the roller.
- Find a suitable vein. Try to avoid the dorsum of the hand and the antecubital fossa.
- Apply the tourniquet to the arm and re-verify the vein.
- Put on the gloves.
- Clean the skin and let it dry.
- Remove the cannula from its packaging and remove its cap.

- Tell the patient to expect a 'sharp scratch'.
- Anchor the vein by stretching the skin and insert the cannula at an angle of approximately 30 degrees.
- Once a flashback is seen, advance the cannula and needle by about 2 mm.
- Pull back slightly on the needle and advance the cannula into the vein.
- Release the tourniquet.
- Press on the vein over the tip of the cannula and remove the needle. Do not cap the cannula.
- Immediately put the needle into the sharps box.
- Attach the giving set.
- Apply the adhesive plaster to fix the cannula.
- Adjust the drip-rate (1 drop per second is equivalent to about 1 litre per 6 hours).

After the procedure

- Ensure that the patient is comfortable.
- Thank the patient.
- Discard any rubbish.
- Sign the fluid chart (if appropriate).

Prescribing intravenous simple fluids (suggested approach for an OSCE station)

1. Inspect the patient for signs of dehydration (e.g. inspect the tongue).
2. Assess the patient's pulse, BP, and JVP.
3. Check the patient's urine output.
4. Check the patient's U&Es.
5. Devise a fluid regimen according to your findings and to the overall clinical situation.
6. Monitor the patient's pulse, BP, JVP, urine output, and U&Es as appropriate for the clinical situation.

Be particularly cautious in the elderly and in those with cardiac or renal failure, and never forget that fluid and electrolyte imbalances can be fatal.

A commonly prescribed 24-hourly fluid regimen for a healthy adult is:

Normal 0.9% saline	1 l		over 8 hours
Normal 0.9% saline	1 l		over 8 hours
5% dextrose	1 l	+ 20 mmol KCl	over 8 hours

The full complexities of fluid prescription (including colloids and blood products) are beyond the scope of this book: please refer to a textbook of internal medicine.

Station 5

Blood transfusion

Specifications: This station requires you either to cannulate an anatomical arm and set up a blood transfusion, or simply to set up a blood transfusion. You may be instructed to talk through parts of the procedure.

Before starting

- Introduce yourself to the patient.
- Explain the requirement for a blood transfusion and ensure that he is consenting.
- Ensure that baseline observations have been recorded (pulse rate, blood pressure, and temperature).

Cannulation

See *Station 4*.

Blood transfusion

1. Sample collection

- Confirm the patient's name and date of birth and check his identity bracelet.
- Extract 10 ml of blood into a pink tube.
- Immediately label the tube and request form with the patient's identifying data: name, date of birth, and hospital number.
- Fill out a blood transfusion form, specifying the total number of units required.
- Ensure that the tube reaches the laboratory promptly.

2. Blood transfusion prescription

- Prescribe the number of units of blood required in the intravenous infusion section of the patient's prescription chart. Each unit of blood should be prescribed separately and be administered over a period of 4 hours.
- If the patient is elderly or has a history of heart failure, consider prescribing 20 mg of oral frusemide with the second and fourth units of blood.
- Arrange for the blood bag to be delivered. The blood transfusion must commence within 30 minutes of the blood leaving the blood refrigerator.

3. Checking procedures

Ask a registered nurse or another doctor to go through the following checking procedures with you:

A. Positively identify the patient by asking him for his name, date of birth, and address.
B. Confirm the patient's identifying data and ensure that they match those on his identity bracelet, case notes, prescription chart, and blood compatibility report.
C. Record the blood group and serial number on the unit of blood and make sure that they match the blood group and serial number on the blood compatibility report and the blood compatibility label attached to the blood unit.
D. Check the expiry date on the unit of blood.
E. Inspect the blood bag for leaks or blood clots or discoloration.

4. Blood administration

- Attach one end of the transfusion giving set to the blood bag and run it through to ensure that any air in the tubing has been expelled.
- Attach the other end of the giving set to the IV cannula.
- Adjust the drip rate so that the unit of blood is administered over 4 hours (1 drop per second is equivalent to about 1 litre per 6 hours).
- Sign the prescription chart and the blood compatibility report recording the date and time the transfusion was commenced. The prescription chart and blood compatibility report should also be signed by your checking colleague.

5. Patient monitoring

- Record the patient's pulse rate, blood pressure, and temperature at 0, 15, and 30 minutes, and then hourly thereafter.
- Ensure that the nursing staff observe the patient for signs of adverse transfusion reactions such as fever, tachycardia, hypotension, urticaria, nausea, chest pain, and breathlessness.

Examiner's questions: complications of blood transfusion	
Immune	Acute haemolytic reaction, (usually due to ABO incompatibility)
	Delayed haemolytic reaction, (usually due to Rhesus, Kell, Duffy, etc., incompatibility)
	Non-haemolytic reactions such as febrile reactions, urticarial reactions, and anaphylaxis
Infectious	Hepatitis
	HIV/AIDS
	Other viral agents
	Bacteria
	Parasites
Cardiovascular	Left ventricular failure from volume overload
Complications of massive transfusion (>10 U)	Hypothermia, coagulopathy, acid–base disturbances, hyperkalaemia, citrate toxicity, iron overload
Other	Air embolism
	Thrombophlebitis

Station 6

Intramuscular, subcutaneous, and intradermal drug injection

Specifications: A model or skin pad in lieu of a patient.

Before starting

- Introduce yourself to the patient.
- Discuss the procedure and obtain consent.
- Gather the appropriate equipment.

The equipment

- Non-sterile gloves.
- Drug.
- Diluent (usually sterile water or saline).
- Appropriately sized syringe (e.g. 1 or 2 ml).
- 21G (green) needle and 23G (blue) or 25G (orange) needle*.

- Alcohol swab.
- Cotton wool.
- Plaster.
- Sharps bin.

*Note that the colour scheme for needles is not the same as that for cannulae (see *Station 4*)

The procedure

- Consult the prescription chart and check:
    - the identity of the patient
    - the prescription: validity, drug, dose, diluent (if appropriate), route of administration, date and time of administration
    - drug allergies, anticoagulation
- Check the doses and expiry dates of the drugs on their vials.
- Wash your hands and don the gloves.
- Attach a 21G needle to the syringe and draw up the correct volume of the drug, making sure you expel any air in the syringe.
- Remove the needle and attach a 23G needle to the syringe for IM/SC administration or a 25G needle for ID administration.
- Ask the patient to expose his upper arm or leg and ensure that the target muscle is completely relaxed.
- Identify landmarks in an attempt to avoid injuring nerves and vessels.
- Clean the exposed site with an alcohol wipe and allow it to dry.

Intramuscular injection technique

- For older children and adults, the densest portion of the deltoid muscle (above the armpit and below the acromion) is the preferred IM injection site. The gluteal muscle is best avoided as the needle may not reach the muscle and there is a risk of damage to the sciatic nerve, not to mention the general embarrassment of the thing. In infants and toddlers, the vastus lateralis muscle in the anterolateral aspect of the middle or upper thigh is the preferred IM injection site.
- With your free hand, slightly stretch the skin at the site of injection.
- Introduce the needle at an 80–90 degree angle to the patient's skin in a quick, firm motion.

Figure 2. Intramuscular, subcutaneous, and intradermal injection techniques.

- Pull on the syringe's plunger to ensure that you have not entered a blood vessel. If you aspirate blood, you need to start again with a new needle, and at a different site.
- Slowly inject the drug and quickly remove the needle.
- Dispose of the needle in the sharps bin.
- If bleeding occurs, apply gentle pressure over the bleeding/injection site with some cotton wool.

Subcutaneous injection technique

- Bunch the skin between thumb and forefinger, thereby lifting the adipose tissue from the underlying muscle.
- Insert the needle at a 45 degree angle in a quick, firm motion.
- Release the skin.
- Pull on the syringe's plunger to ensure that you have not entered a blood vessel.
- Slowly inject the drug.
- Dispose of the needle in the sharps bin.
- Apply gentle pressure over the injection site with some cotton wool.

Intradermal injection technique

- Stretch the skin taut between thumb and forefinger.
- Hold the needle so that the bevel is uppermost.
- Insert the needle at a 15 degree angle, almost parallel to the skin.
- Ensure that the needle is visible beneath the surface of the epidermis.
- Slowly inject the drug.
- A visible bleb should form. If not, immediately withdraw the needle and start again.
- Dispose of the needle in the sharps bin.

After the procedure

- Ensure that the patient is comfortable.
- Sign the prescription chart and record the date, time, drug, dose, and injection site of the injection in the medical records.
- Ensure that the patient is comfortable.
- Ask him if he has any questions or concerns.
- Thank him.

Station 7

Intravenous drug injection

Specifications: An anatomical arm in lieu of a patient. This station is likely to require you to demonstrate and/or talk through the administration of an intravenous (IV) drug with a needle and syringe.

Before starting

- Introduce yourself to the patient and confirm their name and date of birth.
- Discuss the procedure and obtain consent.
- Gather the correct equipment.

The equipment

- Patient's drug chart.
- *British National Formulary.*
- Non-sterile gloves.
- Drug.
- Diluent (usually sterile water).
- Appropriately sized syringes.
- 21G (green) needle (×2).
- Tourniquet.
- Alcohol wipes.
- Cotton wool.
- Pre-filled 5 ml syringe containing saline flush.
- Sharps bin.

The procedure

- Consult the prescription chart and check:
  - the identity of the patient
  - the prescription: validity, drug, dose, diluent (if appropriate), route of administration, date and time of administration
  - drug allergies
- Look in the *BNF* and check the form of the drug, whether it needs reconstituting, the type and volume of diluent required, and the speed of administration.
- Check the name, dose and expiry date of the drug on the vial and the name and expiry date of the diluent.
- Indicate that you would also ask a colleague to confirm the name, dose, and expiry date of the drug and the name and expiry date of the diluent.
- Wash your hands and don the gloves.
- Attach a 21G (green) needle to a syringe and draw up the correct volume of the diluent.
- Reconstitute the drug with the diluent, ensuring that it is completely dissolved.
- Draw up the reconstituted drug into the same syringe.
- Remove the needle and attach a fresh 21G needle to the syringe.
- Apply a tourniquet to the model arm and select a suitable vein.
- Clean the venepuncture site with an alcohol wipe.
- Retract the skin with your non-dominant hand to stabilise the vein and insert the needle into the vein until a flashback is seen.
- Undo the tourniquet.
- Administer the drug at the correct speed.
- Remove the needle from the vein and apply pressure on the puncture site using a piece of cotton wool.
- Dispose of the needle in the sharps bin.
- Remove the gloves and wash your hands.

After the procedure

- Ensure that the patient is comfortable.
- Sign the prescription chart and record the date, time, drug, dose, and injection site of the intravenous injection in the medical records.
- Indicate that you would have your checking colleague countersign it.
- Ensure that the patient is comfortable.
- Ask him if he has any questions or concerns.
- Thank him.

Station 8

Examination of a superficial mass and of lymph nodes

Before starting

- Introduce yourself to the patient.
- Explain the examination and ask him for consent to carry it out.
- Position him appropriately and ensure that he is comfortable.

The examination

- Look at the lump and note its location and any changes to the overlying skin, e.g. inflammation, tethering.
- Ask the patient if the lump is painful before you palpate it. Is the pain only brought on by palpation or is it a more constant pain?
- Palpate the lump in a rotary motion with the pads of your fingers. Does the lump feel warm at first touch? Now consider:
  - number (solitary or multiple)
  - size
  - shape
  - surface (smooth or irregular)
  - consistency (e.g. soft, firm, hard, fluctuant, compressible, rubbery)
  - mobility (fixation)
- Transilluminate the lump by holding between the fingers of one hand and shining a pen torch to it with the other. A bright red glow indicates fluid whereas a dull or absent glow suggests a solid lesion.
- If appropriate, determine whether the lump is pulsatile. This can be done by observing the lump carefully for pulsatile movements, palpating it, and/or auscultating it.
- If appropriate, examine the draining lymph nodes (as shown on the next page).

After examining the lump

- Ask the patient if he has any questions or concerns.
- Thank the patient.
- Summarise your findings and offer a differential diagnosis.
- If appropriate, suggest further investigations, e.g. aspirate, biopsy, ultrasound, CT.

Lymph node examination

Head and neck

The patient should be sitting up and examined from behind. With the fingers of both hands, palpate the submental, submandibular, parotid, and pre- and post-auricular nodes. Next palpate the anterior and posterior cervical nodes and the occipital nodes.

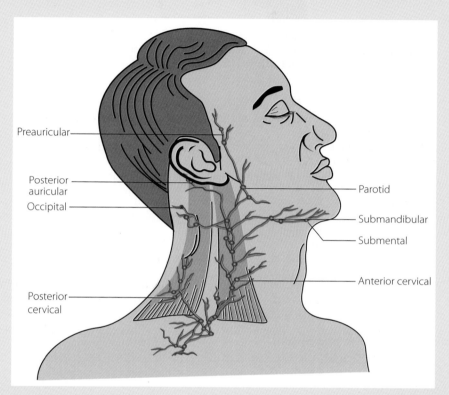

Figure 3. Lymph nodes in the head and neck.

Upper body

- Palpate the supraclavicular and infraclavicular nodes on either side of the clavicle.
- Expose the right axilla by lifting and abducting the arm and supporting it at the wrist with your right hand.
- With your left hand, palpate the following lymph node groups:
  - the apical
  - the anterior
  - the posterior
  - the nodes of the medial aspect of the humerus
- Now expose the left axilla by lifting and abducting the left arm and supporting at the wrist with your left hand.
- With your right hand, palpate the lymph node groups, as listed above.

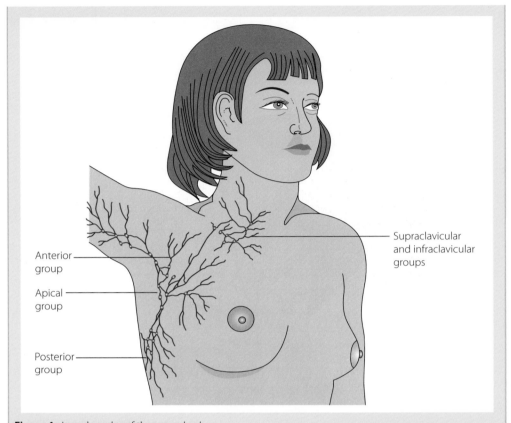

Figure 4. Lymph nodes of the upper body.

Lower body

Palpate the superficial inguinal nodes (horizontal and vertical), which lie below the inguinal ligament and near the great saphenous vein respectively, then the popliteal node in the popliteal fossa.

Chest pain history

Before starting

- Introduce yourself to the patient.
- Explain that you are going to ask him some questions to uncover the nature of his chest pain, and ask for his consent to do this.
- Ensure that he is comfortable; if not, make sure that he is.

The history

- Name, age, occupation, and ethnic origin.

Presenting complaint and history of presenting complaint

- Ask about the nature of the chest pain. Use open questions and give the patient the time to tell his story. Also remember to be empathetic: chest pain can be a very frightening experience.
- Elicit the patient's ideas and concerns.
- For any pain, determine its:
  - site and radiation
  - character
  - severity (e.g. 1 to 10, sleep disturbance)
  - onset and duration
  - aggravating and alleviating factors (exercise, cold air, large meals, alcohol, movement)
  - associated symptoms and signs; ask specifically about nausea and vomiting, shortness of breath, dizziness, cough, and palpitations
- Ask about any previous episodes of chest pain.

Past medical history

- Current, past, and childhood illnesses.
- In particular, ask about coronary heart disease, myocardial infarction, rheumatic fever, stroke, intermittent claudication, hypertension, hyperlipidaemia, diabetes, smoking, and alcohol use.
- Surgery.

Drug history

- Prescribed medication, including the oral contraceptive pill if female.
- Over-the-counter medication.
- Illicit drugs.
- Allergies.

Family history

- Parents, siblings, and children. Ask specifically about heart disease, hypertension, and other heritable cardiovascular risk factors.

Social history

- Effect of the chest pain on the patient's life:
  - employment
  - housing
  - hobbies

After taking the history

- Ask the patient if there is anything else that he might add that you have forgotten to ask. This is an excellent question to ask in clinical practice, and an even better one to ask in exams.
- Thank the patient.
- Summarise your findings and offer a differential diagnosis.
- State that you would like to examine the patient and order some investigations, for example, ECG and chest X-ray, to confirm your diagnosis.

Most common conditions likely to appear in a chest pain history station	
Angina	Pulmonary embolus
Gastro-oesophageal reflux disease	Musculoskeletal complaint
Chest infection	Panic attack
Pleurisy	

 If you cannot differentiate angina from gastro-oesophageal reflux disease, advise a therapeutic trial of an antacid or a nitrate and/or record an ECG.

Cardiovascular risk assessment

Cardiovascular risk factors can usefully be divided into fixed (non-modifiable) and modifiable risk factors. Fixed risk factors include older age, male gender, family history, and a South Asian background. Modifiable risk factors include hypertension, hyperlipidaemia, diabetes, smoking, alcohol, exercise, and stress. Having one or more of these risk factors does not mean that a person is going to develop cardiovascular disease, but merely that he is at increased probability of developing it. Conversely, having no risk factors is not a guarantee that a person is not going to develop cardiovascular disease.

Before starting

- Introduce yourself to the patient.
- Explain that you are going to ask him some questions to assess his risk of cardiovascular disease (coronary heart disease, cerebrovascular disease, vascular disease) and ask for his consent to do this.

 Remember to be tactful in your questioning, and to respond sensitively to the patient's ideas and concerns.

The risk assessment

If this information has not already been provided or disclosed, find out the patient's reason for attending. Then note or enquire about:

Fixed risk factors

1. Age.
2. Sex.
3. Ethnic background. People from a South Asian background are at a notably higher risk of cardiovascular disease.
4. Family history. Ask about a family history of cardiovascular disease and risk factors for cardiovascular disease such as hypertension, hyperlipidaemia and diabetes mellitus.

Modifiable risk factors

5. Hypertension. If hypertensive, ask about latest blood pressure measurement, time since first diagnosis, and any medication being taken.
6. Hyperlipidaemia. If hyperlipidaemic, ask about latest serum cholesterol level, time since first diagnosis, and any medication being taken.
7. Diabetes mellitus. If diabetic, ask about medication being taken, level of diabetes control being achieved, time since first diagnosis, and presence of complications.
8. Cigarette smoking. If a smoker or ex-smoker, ask about number of years spent smoking and average number of cigarettes smoked per day. Does the patient also smoke roll-ups and cannabis?
9. Alcohol. Ask about the number of units of alcohol drunk in a day. Note that depending on the amount and type that is drunk, alcohol can be either a protective factor or a risk factor.
10. Lack of exercise. Ask about amount of exercise taken in a day or week. Does the patient walk to work or walk to the shops?
11. Stress. Ask about occupational history and home life.

Table 2. Desirable lipid levels	
Total cholesterol	≤ 5.0 mmol/l
LDL cholesterol (fasting)	< 3.0 mmol/l
HDL cholesterol	≥ 1.2 mmol/l
Total cholesterol/HDL cholesterol	≤ 4.5
Tryglycerides (fasting)	≤ 1.5 mmol/l

NB. Patients at high risk of cardiovascular disease should aim for even better than these figures.

After the assessment

- If you have time, assess the extent of any cardiovascular disease.
- Ask the patient if there is anything he would like to add that you may have forgotten to ask about.
- Give him feedback on his cardiovascular risk (e.g. low, medium, high), and indicate a further course of action if appropriate (e.g. further investigations or further appointment to discuss reducing modifiable risk factors).
- Address any remaining concerns.

Blood pressure measurement

Before starting

- Introduce yourself to the patient.
- Explain the procedure and ask for his consent to carry it out.
- Tell him that he might feel some discomfort as the cuff is inflated, and that the blood pressure measurement may have to be repeated.

 Avoid white coat hypertension by putting the patient at ease. Briefly discuss a non-threatening subject, such as the patient's journey to the clinic, or the weather.

The procedure

- Position the patient's right arm so that it is horizontal at the level of the mid-sternum.
- Place the vertical column so that it is at eye level.
- Locate the brachial artery at about 2 cm above the antecubital fossa.
- Select an appropriately sized cuff and apply it to the arm, ensuring that it fits securely.
- Inflate the cuff to 20–30 mmHg more than the estimated systolic blood pressure. You can estimate the systolic blood pressure by palpating the brachial or radial artery pulse and inflating the cuff until you can no longer feel it.
- Place the stethoscope over the brachial artery pulse, ensuring that it does not touch the cuff.
- Reduce the pressure in the cuff at a rate of 2–3 mmHg.
- The first consistent Korotkov sounds indicate the systolic blood pressure.
  - The muffling and disappearance of the Korotkov sounds indicate the diastolic blood pressure.
  - Record the blood pressure as the systolic reading over the diastolic reading. Do not attempt to 'round off' your readings; to an examiner's ear, 143/88 usually rings more true than 140/90.
- If the blood pressure is higher than 140/90, indicate that you might take a second reading after giving the patient a one minute rest.

 If the patient has a history of postural hypotension, you must also record the standing blood pressure.

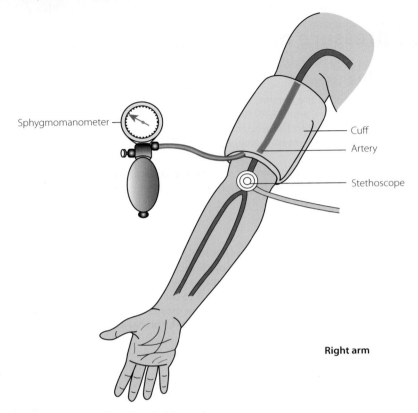

Figure 5. Positioning of the cuff and head of the stethoscope.

After the procedure

- Ensure that the patient is comfortable.
- Tell the patient his blood pressure and explain its significance. Hypertension can only be confirmed by several blood pressure measurements taken over time.
- Thank the patient.

Cardiovascular and respiratory medicine

Examiner's questions

Causes of secondary hypertension:

High catecholamines as in phaeochromocytoma

High glucocorticoids as in Cushing's syndrome

High mineralocorticoids as in Conn's syndrome

Renal disease

Renal artery stenosis

Coarctation of the aorta

Hyper- or hypo-thyroidism

Parahyperthyroidism

Pre-eclampsia

Illicit drugs

Complications of hypertension:

Cerebrovascular accident (haemorrhage or infarct)

Retinopathy

Ischaemic heart disease

Left ventricular failure

Renal failure

Investigations in hypertension:

This involves confirming hypertension, assessing for a possible secondary cause, and assessing for end-organ damage (see above)

Cardiovascular examination

Before starting

- Introduce yourself to the patient.
- Explain the examination and ask for his consent to carry it out.
- Position him at 45 degrees, and ask him to remove his top(s).
- Ensure that he is comfortable.

The examination

General inspection

- From the end of the couch, observe the patient's general appearance (age, state of health, nutritional status, and any other obvious signs). Is the patient breathless or cyanosed?
- Inspect the precordium for the presence of any abnormal pulsation and the chest for any scars. A median sternotomy might have been performed for coronary artery bypass grafting, for valve surgery, or for the repair of a congenital defect. Don't miss a pacemaker if it is there!

Figure 6. Pacemakers can be visible from outside the body.

Reproduced with permission from Julia Freeman-Woolpert (www.sxc.hu/profile/juliaf).

Inspection and examination of the hands

- Take both hands noting:
  - temperature
  - colour
  - the presence of clubbing (endocarditis, cyanotic congenital heart disease)
  - the presence of splinter haemorrhages (subacute infective endocarditis)
  - the presence of nail signs (leukonychia – hypoalbuminaemia, koilonychia – iron deficiency)
- Determine the rate, rhythm, and character of the radial pulse. Take the pulse in both arms to exclude coarctation of the aorta.
- Indicate that you would like to record the blood pressure (see *Station 11*).

Figure 7. Splinter haemorrhage.

Inspection and examination of the head and neck

- Inspect the sclera and conjunctivae for signs of anaemia.
- Inspect the mouth for signs of central cyanosis.
- Assess the jugular venous pressure and the jugular venous pulse form: having asked the patient to turn his head *slightly* to one side, look at the internal jugular vein medial to the clavicular head of sternocleidomastoid. Assuming that the patient is at 45 degrees, the vertical height of the jugular distension from the sternal angle should be no greater than 4 cm.
- Locate the carotid pulse and assess its character.

Height of jugular
venous distention

4 cm

Sternal angle
(angle of Louis)

45°

Figure 8. Assessing the jugular venous pressure.

 Never palpate both carotid pulses simultaneously.

Palpation of the heart

 Ask the patient if he has any chest pain.

- Determine the location and character of the apex beat. It is normally located at the mid-clavicular line, at the level of the fifth intercostal space. A 'tapping' apex beat is likely to indicate mitral stenosis; a 'heaving' apex beat is likely to indicate left ventricular hypertrophy.
- Place your hand over the cardiac apex and on either side of the sternum and feel for any heaves and thrills.

Auscultation of the heart

- Listen for heart sounds, additional sounds, murmurs, and pericardial rub. Using the stethoscope's diaphragm, listen in the:
  - *aortic area*
    right second intercostal space near the sternum
  - *pulmonary area*
    left second intercostal space near the sternum
  - *tricuspid area*
    left third, fourth, and fifth intercostal spaces near the sternum
  - *mitral area*
    left fifth intercostal space, in the mid-clavicular line

Ausculation points

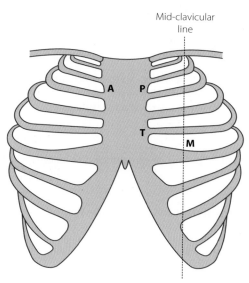

Figure 9. Auscultation points.

- In addition:
  - ask the patient to bend forward and to hold his breath in expiration. Using the stethoscope's diaphragm, listen at the left sternal edge in the fourth intercostal space for the mid-diastolic murmur of aortic regurgitation.
  - ask the patient to turn onto his left side and to hold his breath in expiration. Using the stethoscope's *bell*, listen in the mitral area for the mid-diastolic murmur of mitral stenosis.
  - listen over the carotid arteries for any bruits

Table 3.	Grading murmurs
I	Barely audible murmur
II	Soft and localised murmur
III	Murmur of moderate intensity that is immediately audible
IV	Murmur of loud intensity
V	Murmur of loud intensity with a palpable precordial thrill
VI	As above, except that the murmur is audible even as the stethoscope is lifted from the chest wall

Table 4.	Common conditions associated with murmurs
Aortic stenosis	Slow-rising pulse, heaving cardiac apex, mid-systolic murmur best heard in the aortic area and radiating to the carotids and cardiac apex
Mitral regurgitation	Displaced, thrusting cardiac apex, pan-systolic murmur best heard in the mitral area and radiating to the axilla
Aortic regurgitation	Collapsing pulse, thrusting cardiac apex, diastolic murmur best heard at the left sternal edge
Mitral valve prolapse	Mid-systolic click, late-systolic murmur best heard in the mitral area

Chest examination

- Percuss and auscultate the chest, especially at the bases of the lungs. Heart failure can cause pulmonary oedema and pleural effusions.

Abdominal examination

- Palpate the abdomen to exclude ascites and/or an enlarged liver.
- Check for the presence of an aortic aneurysm.
- Ballot the kidneys and listen for any renal artery bruits.

Ankle oedema

- Test for the dependent or 'pitting' oedema of cardiac failure.

Peripheral pulses

- Feel the temperature of the feet and then palpate the:
  - femoral pulses
  - popliteal pulses
  - posterior tibial pulses
  - dorsalis pedis pulses

After the examination

- Indicate that you would test the urine, examine the retina with an ophthalmoscope and, if appropriate, order some key investigations, e.g. ECG, CXR, echocardiogram.
- Cover the patient up.
- Thank the patient.
- Ensure that he is comfortable.
- Summarise your findings and offer a differential diagnosis.

Most common conditions likely to come up in a cardiovascular examination station
Murmurs (see *Table 4*)
Heart failure
Median sternotomy scar
Pacemaker

Peripheral vascular system examination

In this station you may be asked to restrict your examination to the arterial or venous system only. You must therefore be able to separate out the signs for either (see *Table 6*).

Before starting

- Introduce yourself to the patient.
- Explain the examination and ask for his consent to carry it out.
- Expose his legs, including his feet.

The examination

Inspection

- Skin changes: pallor, shininess, loss of body hair, *atrophie blanche* (ivory-white areas), pigmentation, inflammation, eczema.
- Thickened dystrophic nails.
- Scars.
- Signs of gangrene: blackened skin, nail infection, amputated toes.
- Venous and arterial ulcers. Remember to look in the interdigital spaces.
- Oedema.
- Varicose veins (ask the patient to stand up). Varicose veins are often associated with incompetent valves in the long and short saphenous veins.

 Do not make the common mistake of asking the patient to stand up before having examined for varicose veins.

Palpation and special tests

- Skin temperature. Compare both legs.
- Capillary refill. Compress a nail bed for 5 seconds and let go. It should take less than 2 seconds for the nail bed to return to its normal colour.
  - Peripheral pulses.
  - Femoral pulse at the inguinal ligament.
  - Popliteal pulse in the popliteal space (flex the knee).
  - Posterior tibial pulse behind the medial malleolus.
  - *Dorsalis pedis* pulse over the dorsum of the foot, just lateral to the extensor tendon of the great toe.
- Buerger's test:
  - lift both of the patient's legs to a 45 degree angle and note the change in skin colour
  - ask the patient to dangle his legs over the edge of the couch; if the arterial supply is normal, the original skin colour should return in less than 10 seconds
- Oedema. Firm 'non-pitting' oedema is a sign of chronic venous insufficiency (compare to the 'pitting' oedema of cardiac failure).
- Varicose veins. Tenderness on palpation suggests thrombophlebitis.
- Trendelenburg's test:
  - elevate the leg to 90 degrees to drain the veins of blood
  - apply a tourniquet to the upper thigh

- ask the patient to stand up – the veins should gradually fill up in 30–35 seconds
- release the tourniquet: sudden additional filling of the veins is a sign of sapheno-femoral incompetence

Auscultation

- Femoral arteries.
- Abdominal aorta.

After the examination

- Thank the patient.
- Ensure that he is comfortable.
- Summarise your findings and offer a differential diagnosis.

Table 5. Examination of the arterial or venous system only	
Arterial system	**Venous system**
Pallor	*Atrophie blanche*
Shininess	Pigmentation
Dystrophic nails	Inflammation
Loss of body hair	Eczema
Arterial ulcers	Oedema (non-pitting)
Signs of gangrene	Venous ulcers
Skin temperature	Varicose veins
Capillary refill	Scars due to varicose vein surgery
Peripheral pulses	Trendelenburg test
Buerger's test	Perthes' test (if after the gold medal)
Auscultation of femoral arteries and aorta	
ABPI (if time permits, see *Station 14*)	

Figure 10. Large venous ulcer. Arterial and neuropathic ulcers tend to be on the sole of the foot and on pressure points, and venous ulcers on the medial and lateral aspects of the leg, above the malleoli.

Reproduced from *BMJ* (2000) **320:** 1589–91, with permission.

Ankle-brachial pressure index (ABPI)

Specifications: You are most likely to be requested to measure the ABPI for one arm and ankle only.

Calculating and interpreting ABPI

Right arm systolic pressure

Left arm systolic pressure

Right ankle systolic pressure — Posterior tibial / Dorsalis pedis

Posterior tibial / Dorsalis pedis — Left ankle systolic pressure

Right ABPI

$$\frac{\text{Higher of the two right ankle pressures}}{\text{Higher of the two arm pressures}}$$

Left ABPI

$$\frac{\text{Higher of the two left ankle pressures}}{\text{Higher of the two arm pressures}}$$

Figure 11. Calculating ABPI.

Table 6. ABPI interpretation	
ABPI	**Interpretation**
> 0.95	Normal
0.5–0.9	Claudication pain
< 0.5	Rest pain
< 0.2	Ulceration and gangrene

Before starting

- Introduce yourself to the patient.
- Explain the procedure and ask him for consent to carry it out.
- Position him at 45° with his sleeves and trousers rolled up.
- Ensure that he is comfortable.
- State that you would allow him 5 minutes resting time before taking measurements.

The procedure

Brachial systolic pressure

- Place an appropriately sized cuff around the arm, as for any blood pressure recording.
- Locate the brachial pulse by palpation and apply contact gel at this site.
- Angle the hand-held Doppler probe at 45° to the skin and locate the best possible signal. Apply only gentle pressure, or else you risk occluding the artery.
- Inflate the cuff until the signal disappears.
- Progressively deflate the cuff and record the pressure at which the signal reappears.
- Repeat the procedure for the other arm or state that you would do so.
- Retain the higher of the two readings.

 Take care not to allow the probe to slide away from the line of the artery.

Ankle systolic pressure

- Place an appropriately sized cuff around the ankle immediately above the malleoli.
- Locate the dorsalis pedis pulse by palpation or with the hand-held Doppler probe and apply contact gel at this site.
- Angle the hand-held Doppler probe at 45° to the skin and locate the best possible signal. Apply only gentle pressure, or else you risk occluding the artery.
- Inflate the cuff until the signal disappears.
- Progressively deflate the cuff, and record the pressure at which the signal reappears.
- Repeat the procedure for the posterior tibial pulse, which is posterior and inferior to the medial malleolus.
- Repeat the procedure for the dorsalis pedis and posterior tibial pulses of the other ankle or state that you would do so.
- For each ankle, retain the higher of the two readings.

After the procedure

- Clean the patient's skin of contact gel and allow him time to restore his clothing.
- Clean the hand-held Doppler probe of contact gel.
- Wash your hands.
- Calculate the ABPI and explain its significance to the patient.
- Ask the patient if he has any questions or concerns.
- Thank the patient.

Breathlessness history

Before starting

- Introduce yourself to the patient.
- Explain that you are going to ask him some questions to uncover the nature of his breathlessness, and ask for his consent to do this.
- Ensure that he is comfortable; if not, make sure that he is.

The history

- Name, age, and occupation.

Presenting complaint

- Ask about the nature of the breathlessness. Use open questions.
- Elicit the patient's ideas and concerns.

History of presenting complaint

Ask about:

- Onset, duration, and variability of breathlessness.
- Provoking and relieving factors.
- Associated symptoms (wheeze, stridor, cough, sputum, haemoptysis, fever, night sweats, anorexia, loss of weight, chest pain, dizziness).
- Severity (exercise tolerance, sleep disturbance – orthopnoea, paroxysmal nocturnal dyspnoea).
- Previous episodes of breathlessness.
- Smoking.

Past medical history

- Current, past, and childhood illnesses. Ask specifically about atopy (asthma/eczema/hay fever), pneumonia, bronchitis, and tuberculosis.
- Previous investigations (e.g. bronchoscopy, chest X-ray).
- Surgery.

Drug history

- Prescribed medication (especially bronchodilators, NSAIDs, β-blockers, ACE inhibitors, amiodarone, and steroids).
- Over-the-counter medication.
- Recreational drugs.
- Allergies.

Family history

- Parents, siblings, and children. Focus especially on respiratory diseases such as atopy, cystic fibrosis, tuberculosis, and emphysema (α1-antitrypsin deficiency).

Social history

- Employment, past and present. Ask about occupational exposure (mining, farming, asbestos).
- Housing.
- Travel, tuberculosis contacts.
- Use of alcohol.
- Hobbies (especially pigeons and budgerigars).

After taking the history

- Ask the patient if there is anything else he might add that you have forgotten to ask.
- Thank the patient.
- Summarise your findings and offer a differential diagnosis.
- State that you would like to examine the patient and carry out some investigations to confirm your diagnosis.

Most common conditions likely to appear in a breathlessness history station	
Asthma	Lung cancer
Pneumonia	Tuberculosis
Pleural effusion	Heart failure
Chronic obstructive pulmonary disease	Panic attack
Pulmonary embolism	

Respiratory system examination

Before starting

- Introduce yourself to the patient.
- Explain the examination and ask for his consent to carry it out.
- Position him at 45°, and ask him to remove his top(s).
- Ensure that he is comfortable.

The examination

General inspection

- From the end of the couch, observe the patient's general appearance (age, state of health, nutritional status, and any other obvious signs). In particular, is he breathless or cyanosed? Does he have to sit up to breathe? Is his breathing audible? Is he coughing?
- Note:
    - the rate, depth, and regularity of the patient's breathing
    - any deformities of the chest (barrel chest, *pectus excavatum*, *pectus carinatum*) and spine
    - any asymmetry of chest expansion
    - the use of accessory muscles of respiration
    - the presence of operative scars

Figure 12. Respiratory system examination: *pectus excavatum*.

Inspection and examination of the hands

- Take both hands and assess them for colour and temperature.
- Look for clubbing.
- Determine the rate, rhythm, and character of the radial pulse. Is it the bounding pulse of carbon dioxide retention?
- Test for asterixis, the flapping tremor of carbon dioxide retention, by asking the patient to extend both arms with the wrists dorsiflexed and the palms facing forwards.

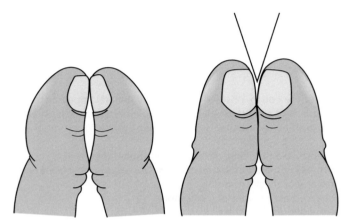

Figure 13. Clubbing. When the dorsum of a finger from one hand is opposed to the dorsum of a finger from the other hand, a diamond shaped window is formed at the base of the nailbeds. In clubbing, this diamond shaped window is obliterated, and a distal angle is created between the fingers.

Figure 14. Finger clubbing.

Reproduced from www.mevis-research.de with permission.

Table 7. The principal causes of clubbing

Respiratory causes	Gastrointestinal causes
Carcinoma	Cirrhosis
Fibrosing alveolitis	Ulcerative colitis
Chronic suppurative lung disease	Crohn's disease
Cardiac causes	Coeliac disease
Infective endocarditis	**Familial**
Cyanotic heart disease	

Table 8. The principal causes of asterixis

Hepatic failure

Renal failure

Cardiac failure

Respiratory failure

Electrolyte abnormalities (hypoglycaemia, hypokalaemia, hypomagnesaemia)

Drug intoxication, e.g. alcohol, phenytoin

CNS causes

Inspection and examination of the head and neck

- Inspect the sclera and conjunctivae for signs of anaemia.
- Inspect the mouth for signs of central cyanosis.
- Assess the jugular venous pressure and the jugular venous pulse form (*cor pulmonale* – right-sided heart failure).
- Palpate the cervical, supraclavicular, infraclavicular, and axillary lymph nodes.

Palpation of the chest

 Ask the patient if he has any chest pain.

- Palpate for tracheal deviation by placing the index and middle fingers of one hand on either side of the trachea in the suprasternal notch. Alternatively, place the index and annular fingers of one hand on either clavicular head and use your middle finger (called the *vulgaris* in Latin) to palpate the trachea.
- Palpate for the position of the cardiac apex.

[Note] Carry out all subsequent steps on the front of the chest and, once this is done, repeat them on the back of the chest. This is much more elegant than to keep on asking the patient to bend forwards and backwards like a Jack-in-the-box.

- Palpate for equal chest expansion, comparing one side to the other. Reduced unilateral chest expansion might be caused by pneumonia, pleural effusion, pneumothorax, and lung collapse. If there is a measuring tape, measure the chest expansion.
- Test for tactile fremitus by placing the flat of the hands on the chest and asking the patient to say 'ninety-nine'. Any other numbers are at your own risk and peril.

Percussion of the chest

- Percuss the chest. Start at the apex of one lung, and compare one side to the other. Do not forget to percuss over the clavicles and on the sides of the chest. For any one area, is the resonance increased (emphysema, pneumothorax) or decreased (consolidation, fibrosis, fluid)?

Auscultation of the chest

- Ask the patient to take deep breaths through the mouth and, using the diaphragm of the stethoscope, auscultate the chest. Start at the apex of one lung, and compare one side to the other. Are the breath sounds vesicular or bronchial? Are there any other added signs?
- Test for vocal resonance by asking the patient to say, 'ninety nine'. If you have already tested for tactile fremitus, it is not necessary to test for vocal resonance.
- Different breath sounds, including the ever elusive whispering pectoriloquy, can be listened to on the University of Loyola's website at: www.meddean.luc.edu/lumen/MedEd/medicine/pulmonar/pd/auditory.htm.

After the examination

- Indicate that you would like to look at the sputum pot, measure the PEFR (see *Station 17*) and, if appropriate, order some key investigations, e.g. a CXR, FBC, CRP, etc.
- Cover the patient up.
- Thank the patient.
- Ensure that he is comfortable.
- Summarise your findings and offer a differential diagnosis.

Most common conditions likely to appear in a respiratory examination station
Chronic and relatively stable chest conditions such:
• Chronic obstructive pulmonary disease
• Cryptogenic fibrosing alveolitis
• Lobectomy

PEFR meter explanation

 Read in conjunction with Station 110: Explaining skills.

Before starting

- Introduce yourself to the patient.
- Check his understanding of asthma.
- Explain the importance of using a PEFR (Peak Expiratory Flow Rate) meter and the importance of using it correctly.
- Explain that the PEFR meter is to be used first thing in the morning and at any time he has symptoms of asthma.

Explain the use of a PEFR meter

Demonstrate and ask the patient to:

- Attach a clean mouthpiece to the meter.
- Slide the marker to the bottom of the numbered scale.
- Stand or sit up straight.
- Hold the peak flow meter horizontal, keeping his fingers away from the marker.
- Take as deep a breath as possible and hold it.
- Insert the mouthpiece into his mouth, sealing his lips around the mouthpiece.
- Exhale as hard as possible into the meter.
- Read and record the meter reading.
- Repeat the procedure three to six times, keeping only the highest score.
- Check this score against the peak flow chart or his previous readings.
- Check the patient's understanding by asking him to carry out the procedure.
- Ask him if he has any questions or concerns.

Interpret a PEFR reading

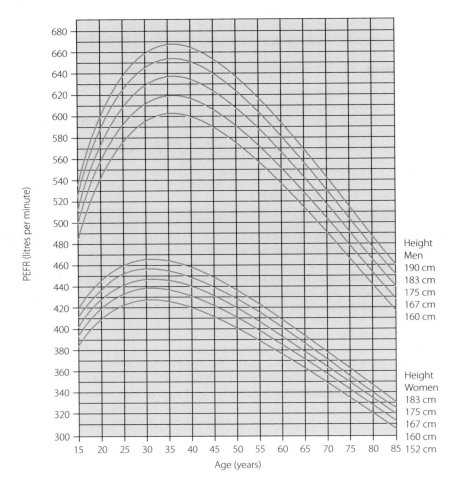

Figure 15. Expected peak flow rates in litres per minute according to age, sex, and height.

Inhaler explanation

 Read in conjunction with Station 110: Explaining skills.

Before starting

- Introduce yourself to the patient.
- Check his understanding of asthma.
- Explain that an inhaler device delivers aerosolised bronchodilator medication for inhalation and that, if used correctly, provides fast and efficient relief from bronchospasm (or airway irritation and narrowing). Furthermore, it is relatively free of systemic side-effects.

Instruct on the use of an inhaler

Demonstrate and ask the patient to:

- Vigorously shake the inhaler.
- Remove the cap from the mouthpiece.
- Hold the inhaler between index finger and thumb.
- Place the inhaler upright about 3–5 cm in front of his mouth.
- Breathe out completely.
- Breathe in deeply, and simultaneously activate the inhaler.
- Close his mouth and hold his breath for 10 seconds and then breathe out.
- Repeat the procedure after 1 minute if relief is insufficient.
- Check his understanding by asking him to carry out the procedure.
- Ask him if he has any questions or concerns.

 If the patient has difficulty co-ordinating breathing in and inhaler activation, he may benefit from the added use of an aerochamber inhaler spacer.

Drug administration via a nebuliser

A nebuliser transforms a drug solution into a fine mist for inhalation via a mouthpiece or face mask. Drugs used in nebulisers include bronchodilators, corticosteroids, and antibiotics (e.g. colistin).

Before starting

- Introduce yourself to the patient.
- Explain the need for a nebuliser and the procedure involved, and ensure consent.
- Explain the drug in the nebuliser and its common side-effects.

The equipment

- An air compressor and tubing.
- A nebuliser cup.
- A mouthpiece or mask.
- A syringe.

- Drug or drug solution (e.g. salbutamol 2.5 ml) in a vial.
- Diluent (e.g. sodium chloride 0.9%) if needed.

Figure 16. Nebuliser set-up.

The procedure

- Consult the prescription chart and check:
  - the identity of the patient
  - the prescription: validity, drug, dose, diluent, route of administration, date and time of starting
  - drug allergies
- Check the name, dose, and expiry date of the drug on the vial.
- Ask a colleague (registered nurse or doctor) to confirm the name, dose, and expiry date of the drug on the vial.
- Place the air compressor on a sturdy surface and plug it into the mains.

As the compressor unit delivers a set airflow rate that is most suitable for asthmatic patients, it should not be used in COPD patients. For COPD patients, connect the tubing to the oxygen outlet in the wall and set the flow rate to 8 l/min.

- Wash your hands.
- Open the vial of drug solution by twisting off the top.
- With the syringe, carefully draw up the correct amount of drug solution.
- Remove the top part of the nebuliser cup and place the drug solution into it.
- Re-attach the top part of the nebuliser cup and connect the mouthpiece or face mask to the nebuliser cup.
- Connect the tubing from the air compressor to the bottom of the nebuliser cup.
- Switch on the air compressor.
- Ask the patient to sit up straight.
- If using a mouthpiece, ask him to clasp it between his teeth and to seal his lips around it. If using a mask, position it comfortably and securely over his face.
- Ask him to take slow, deep breaths through the mouth and, if possible, to hold each breath for 2–3 seconds before breathing out.
- Continue until there is no drug left and the nebuliser begins to splutter (about 10 minutes).
- Turn the compressor off.
- Ask the patient to take several deep breaths and to cough up any secretions.
- Ask him to rinse his mouth with water.
- Wash your hands.

 Should the patient feel dizzy, he should interrupt the treatment and rest for about 5 minutes. After resuming the treatment, he should be instructed to breathe more slowly through the mouthpiece.

After the procedure

- Tell the examiner that you would clean and disinfect the equipment.
- Sign the drug chart and record the diluent used, and the date, time, and dose of the drug in the medical records.
- Indicate that you would have your checking colleague countersign it.
- Ask the patient if he has any questions or concerns.
- Ensure that he is comfortable.

Station 20

Abdominal pain history

Before starting

- Introduce yourself to the patient.
- Explain that you are going to ask him some questions to uncover the cause of his abdominal pain, and ask for his consent to do this.
- Ensure that he is comfortable.

 Ensure that the patient is nil by mouth. Acute abdomen is a surgical complaint and the patient must therefore be kept nil by mouth until the need for surgery has been excluded.

The history

- Name, age, and occupation.

Presenting complaint and history of presenting complaint

- Ask about the nature of the abdominal pain. Use open questions.
- For any pain, try to determine:
  - nature
  - site
  - onset
  - duration
  - radiation
  - aggravating and alleviating factors
  - associated symptoms and signs
- In addition ask about:
  - fever
  - loss of weight or anorexia
  - dysphagia
  - indigestion
  - nausea, vomiting, and haematemesis
  - diarrhoea or constipation
  - melaena or rectal bleeding
  - steatorrhoea
  - jaundice
  - genitourinary symptoms: frequency, dysuria, haematuria
  - menses (menarche, menopause, length of menstrual periods, amount of bleeding, pain, intermenstrual bleeding, last menstrual period)

Past medical history

- Previous episodes of abdominal pain.
- Current, past, and childhood illnesses.
- Surgery.

GI medicine and urology

Drug history

- Prescribed medications. Ask specifically about corticosteroids, NSAIDs, antibiotics, and the contraceptive pill.
- Over-the-counter medication.
- Recreational drugs.
- Allergies.

Family history

- Parents, siblings, and children. Ask specifically about colon cancer, irritable bowel syndrome, inflammatory bowel disease, jaundice, peptic ulcer, and polyps.

Social history

- Alcohol consumption.
- Smoking.
- Travel.
- Employment, past and present.
- Housing.
- Contact with jaundiced patients.

After taking the history

- Ask the patient if there is anything that he might add that you have forgotten to ask.
- Ask the patient if he has any questions or concerns.
- Thank the patient.
- State that you would carry out a full abdominal examination and order some key investigations such as urinalysis, serum analysis, and an abdominal X-ray, as appropriate.
- Summarise your findings and offer a differential diagnosis.

Most common conditions likely to appear in a abdominal pain history station	
Appendicitis	Acute pancreatitis
Gastro-oesophageal reflux disease	Ureteric colic
Peptic ulceration	Diverticulitis
Biliary colic	Colon cancer
Acute cholecystitis	Irritable bowel syndrome

 Remember that basal pneumonia, diabetic ketoacidosis, and an inferior myocardial infarct can also present as abdominal pain.

Station 21

Abdominal examination

Before starting

- Introduce yourself to the patient.
- Ask the patient for permission to examine his abdomen.
- Say to the examiner that you would normally expose the patient from nipples to knees, but that in this case you are going to limit yourself to exposing the patient to the groins.
- Position the patient so that he is lying flat on the couch, with his arms at his side and his head supported by a pillow.
- Ensure that the patient is comfortable.

The examination

General inspection

- From the end of the couch, observe the patient's general appearance (age, state of health, nutritional status, and any other obvious signs).
- Inspect the abdomen for its contours and any obvious distension, localised masses, scars, and skin changes. Ask the patient to lift his head to tense the abdominal muscles.

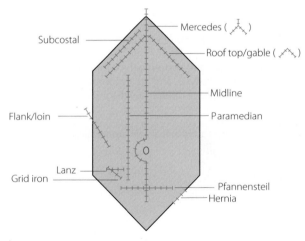

Figure 17. Abdominal scars.

Inspection and examination of the hands

- Take both hands, looking for:
  - clubbing
  - palmar erythema (liver disease)
  - Dupuytren's contracture (cirrhosis)
  - nail signs (leukonychia – hypoalbuminaemia, koilonychia – iron deficiency)
- Test for asterixis or 'liver flap' (hepatic failure) by showing the patient how to extend both arms with the wrists dorsiflexed and the palms facing forwards.

Figure 18. Koilonychia.
Reproduced from www.dermnet.com with permission.

Figure 19. Leukonychia.
Reproduced from http://commons.wikimedia.org with permission.

Figure 20. Dupuytren's contracture.

Inspection and examination of the head, neck, and upper body

- Inspect the sclera and conjunctivae for signs of jaundice or anaemia.
- Inspect the mouth, looking for ulcers (Crohn's disease), angular stomatitis (nutritional defi-ciency), atrophic glossitis (iron deficiency, vitamin B12 deficiency, folate deficiency), furring of the tongue (loss of appetite), and the state of the dentition.
- Examine the neck for lymphadenopathy.
- Examine the upper body for gynaecomastia (cirrhosis), caput medusae, and spider naevi (chronic liver disease).

Figure 21. Atrophic glossitis. Note the loss of filliform papillae.

Reproduced from www.joplink.net – photograph by Dr Echenique-Eligondo.

Palpation of the abdomen

 Ask the patient if he has any abdominal pain and fix upon his face as you palpate his abdomen. Palpate with the palmar surface of your fingers whilst sitting or kneeling beside the patient.

- *Light palpation* – Begin by examining the segment furthest away from any pain or discomfort and systematically palpate the four quadrants and the umbilical area. Look for tenderness, guarding, and any masses.
- *Deep palpation* – For greater precision. Describe and localise any masses.

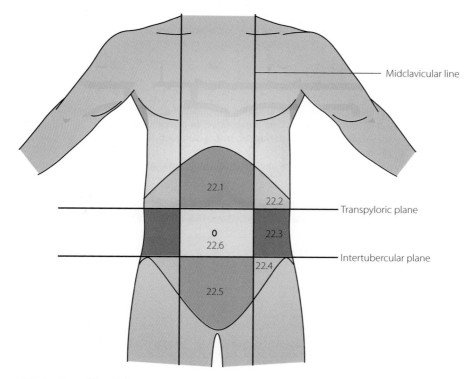

Figure 22. Regions of the abdomen.
22.1 Epigastric
22.2 Left hypochondriac
22.3 Right lumbar
22.4 Right iliac fossa
22.5 Suprapubic/hypogastric
22.6 Umbilical

Palpation of the organs

- *Liver* – Ask the patient to breathe in and out and, starting in the *right lower quadrant*, feel for the liver edge using the flat of your hand or the tips of your fingers. The liver edge, if felt, can be described in terms of regularity, nodularity, and tenderness.
- *Gallbladder* – Palpate for tenderness over the gallbladder region that is at the tip of the right ninth rib.

- *Spleen* – Palpate for the spleen as for the liver, again starting in the *right lower quadrant.*
- *Kidneys* – Position the patient close to the edge of the bed and ballot each kidney using the technique of deep bimanual palpation, which some students do find quite tricky.
- *Aorta* – Palpate the descending aorta between the thumb and the index of your right hand at a point midway between the xiphisternum and the umbilicus.

Percussion

- Percuss the liver area, also remembering to detect its upper border (usually found in the fourth intercostal space).
- Percuss the suprapubic area for undue dullness (bladder distension).
- If the abdomen appears distended, test for shifting dullness (ascites). *Shifting dullness can be tested for by percussing down the right side of the abdomen. If an area of dullness is detected, keep two fingers on it and ask the patient to roll over to his left. Re-percuss the area which should now sound tympanic.*

Auscultation

- Auscultate in the mid-abdomen for abdominal sounds. Listen for 30 seconds before concluding that they are normal, hyperactive, hypoactive, or absent.
- Listen over the abdominal aorta for aortic bruits suggestive of arteriosclerosis or an aneurysm.
- Listen for renal artery bruits 2.5 cm above and lateral to the umbilicus – a bruit suggests renal artery stenosis.

Table 9. Principal causes of altered bowel sounds	
Hypoactive	Constipation
	Drugs such as anticholinergics and opiates
	General anaesthesia
	Abdominal surgery
	Paralytic ileus (absent bowel sounds)
Hyperactive	Diarrhoea of any cause
	Inflammatory bowel disease
	GI bleeding
	Mechanical bowel obstruction (high pitched bowel sounds)

 The following are not usually performed in an abdominal examination station, but they should nevertheless be mentioned at this stage.

Examination of the groins and genitals

(See *Stations 23* and *26*.)

Rectal examination

(See *Station 22*.)

GI medicine and urology

After the examination

- Cover the patient up.
- Thank the patient.
- Ask the patient if he has any questions or concerns.
- State that you would test the urine and order some key investigations, e.g. ultrasound scan, FBC, LFTs, U&Es, and clotting screen.
- Summarise your findings and offer a differential diagnosis.

Most common conditions likely to appear in an abdominal examination station	
Chronic liver disease	Renal transplant
Splenomegaly	Scars
Polycystic kidney	Hernias

Station 22

Rectal examination

Rectal examination is commonly indicated in cases of rectal or GI bleeding (suspected or actual), severe constipation, faecal or urinary incontinence, anal or rectal pain, suspected enlargement of the prostate gland, and urethral discharge or bleeding. It can also be used to screen for cancers of the rectum, colon, and prostate.

Specifications: A plastic model in lieu of a patient.

Before starting

- Introduce yourself to the patient.
- Explain the procedure to him, emphasising that it might be uncomfortable but that it should not be painful, and ask for his consent to carry it out.
- Ask for a chaperone.
- Ask the patient to lower his trousers and underpants.
- Ask him to lie on his left side, to bring his buttocks to the side of the couch, and to bring his knees up to his chest.

The examination

- Put on a pair of gloves.
- Gently separate the buttocks and inspect the anus and surrounding skin. In particular, look out for skin tags, excoriations, ulcers, fissures, prolapsed haemorrhoids, and mucosal prolapse.
- Lubricate the index finger of your right hand.
- Position the finger over the anus, as if pointing to the genitalia.
- Gently insert the finger into the anus, through the anal canal, and into the rectum (Figure 23).

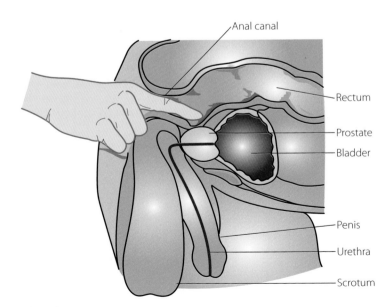

Figure 23. Digital rectal examination.

- Test anal tone by asking the patient to squeeze your finger.
- Rotate the finger so as to palpate the entire circumference of the anal canal and rectum. Feel for any masses, ulcers, or induration.
    - In males pay specific attention to the size, surface, and consistency of the prostate gland.
    - In females, the cervix can usually be palpated.
- Remove the finger and examine the glove. In particular look at the colour of any stool, and for the presence of any mucous or blood.
- Remove and dispose of the gloves.

After the examination

- Clean off any lubricant or faeces on the anus or anal margin.
- Give the patient time to put his clothes back on.
- Ensure that he is comfortable.
- Address any questions or concerns that he may have.
- Present your findings to the examiner, and offer a differential diagnosis.

Station 23

Hernia examination

Inguinal anatomy

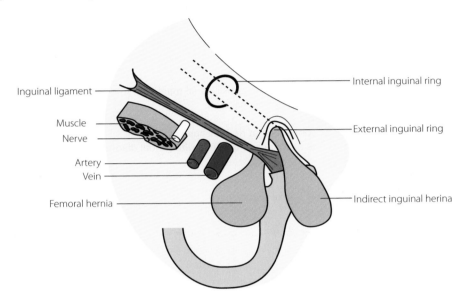

Internal inguinal ring

Inguinal ligament

Muscle

Nerve

Artery

Vein

Femoral hernia

External inguinal ring

Indirect inguinal herina

Figure 24. The inguinal canal runs along the inguinal ligament, from the internal (deep) ring to the external (superficial) ring. The inguinal ligament stretches from the anterior superior iliac spine to the pubic tubercle. The internal ring lies approximately 1.5 cm superior to the femoral pulse, itself in the midline of the inguinal ligament. The external ring lies immediately superior and medial to the pubic tubercle.

Definition of a hernia

A hernia is defined as the protrusion of an organ or part thereof through a deficiency in the wall of the cavity in which it is contained. There are many different types of hernia but the ones that are most likely to be examined and discussed in an OSCE are indirect and direct inguinal hernias and femoral hernias. Their principal differentiating features are summarised in Table 11. The differential diagnosis of a lump in the groin is listed in Table 12.

Table 10. Principal differentiating features of indirect and direct inguinal hernias and femoral hernias		
Indirect hernia	**Direct hernia**	**Femoral hernia**
Neck of hernia is superior to the inguinal ligament/pubic tubercle and lateral to the inferior epigastric vessels	Neck of hernia is superior to the inguinal ligament/ pubic tubercle and medial to the inferior epigastric vessels	Neck of hernia is inferior and lateral to the inguinal ligament pubic tubercle
Accounts for 80% of inguinal hernias	Accounts for 20% of inguinal hernias	Is more common in females
Irreducible	Easily reducible	Often irreducible
Can strangulate	Rarely strangulates	Frequently strangulates

Table 11. Differential diagnosis of a lump in the groin

Superior to the inguinal ligament	Inferior to the inguinal ligament
Indirect or direct inguinal hernia	Femoral hernia
Incisional hernia	Lymph node
Sebaceous cyst	Sebaceous cyst
Lipoma	Lipoma
Undescended testis	Saphena varix
	Femoral artery aneurysm
	Psoas abscess (rare)
	Undescended testis
	Scrotal mass (see *Station 26*)

Before starting

- Introduce yourself to the patient.
- Explain the examination and ask for his consent to carry it out.
- Ask for a chaperone.
- Ask the patient to lie on the couch and to expose his abdomen from the umbilicus to the knees.
- Ensure that he is comfortable.
- Warm up your hands.

 Ensure the patient's dignity at all times.

The examination

Inspection and palpation

- Inspect the groins (both sides!) for an obvious lump. If a lump is visible, determine its location in relation to its surrounding anatomical landmarks. Also determine its size, shape, colour, consistency, and mobility. Is it tender to touch? Can it be transilluminated? (See *Station 8: Examination of a superficial mass*.)
- Look for old surgical scars (incisional hernia).
- Ask the patient to stand up and look again.

Cough impulse and cough tests

(The patient is still standing.)

- Ask the patient to cough and look again.
- Test the lump for a cough impulse. Place two fingers over the lump and ask the patient to cough once more.
- If you are satisfied that the lump is an inguinal hernia, ask the patient to reduce the lump. Once the lump is fully reduced, place two fingers over the internal ring and ask the patient to cough.
  - If the lump does not reappear it is an indirect inguinal hernia. Release your fingers and ask the patient to cough again.
  - If the lump reappears medially it is a direct inguinal hernia.

- Once again ask the patient to reduce the lump. This time place two fingers over the *external* ring and ask the patient to cough.
  - If the lump does not reappear it is a direct inguinal hernia. Release your fingers and ask the patient to cough again.
  - If the lump reappears laterally it is an indirect inguinal hernia.

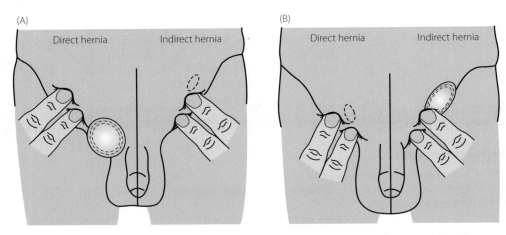

Figure 25. The cough test with two fingers over the internal ring (A) and then over the external ring (B).

After the examination

- Indicate that you would also examine the femoral pulses, inguinal lymph nodes, and scrotum.
- Cover up the patient.
- Ensure that he is comfortable.
- Thank him.
- Summarise your findings and offer a differential diagnosis. Don't fret over your diagnosis as even experienced surgeons are notoriously poor at differentiating between indirect and direct inguinal hernias. Apart from inguinal and femoral hernias, other (more rare) types of hernia are epigastric hernias that occur in the epigastric area in the midline, spigellian or semilunar hernias that occur on the outer border of the rectus muscles, umbilical and paraumbilical hernias that occur at or around the navel, and incisional hernias that occur at the site of an old surgical incision.
- Wash your hands.

Nasogastric intubation

Specifications: A mannequin in lieu of a patient.

Choice of NG tube

Nasogastric (NG or Ryle's) tubes can be used for feeding or drug administration, to decompress the stomach, to obtain a sample of gastric fluid, or to drain the stomach's contents (e.g. after an overdose or if emergency surgery is required). If the tube is being used for aspiration or drainage, a gauge of 10 or greater is required. If not, a fine bore tube should be preferred.

The equipment

- A pair of non-sterile gloves.
- An NG tube of appropriate size.
- K-Y jelly.
- Xylocaine spray.
- A glass of water (if appropriate).
- Tape.
- Stethoscope.
- A 20 ml syringe and some pH paper.
- A spigot or catheter bag.
- A vomit bowl.

Before starting

- Introduce yourself to the patient.
- Explain the need for an NG tube and the procedure for inserting it, and ensure consent.
- Position the patient upright and ask about nostril preference/examine the nostrils.
- Ensure that the patient is comfortable.
- Wash your hands and don the gloves.

The procedure

- Measure the length of NG tube to be inserted by placing the tip of the tube at the nostril and extending the tube behind the ear and then to two fingerbreadths above the umbilicus.
- Lubricate the tip of the NG tube with K-Y jelly.
- Spray the back of the throat with xylocaine or state that you would do so.
- Insert the NG tube into the preferred nostril and slide it along the floor of the nose into the nasopharynx.
- Ask the patient to swallow some water as you continue to advance the tube through the pharynx and oesophagus and into the stomach.
- If the patient coughs or gags, slightly withdraw the tube and leave him some time to recover.
- Insert the tube to the required length.
- Ensure that the tip of the tube is in the stomach.
  - Inject 20 ml of air into the tube and listen over the epigastrium with your stethoscope.
  - Pull back on the plunger to aspirate stomach contents. Test the aspirate with pH paper to confirm its acidity (pH < 6). If a fine-bore tube has been inserted, it may not be possible to aspirate stomach contents.
  - Request a chest X-ray or indicate that you would do so.
- Tape the tube to the nose and to the side of the face.
- Attach a spigot or catheter bag to the NG tube.

After the procedure

- Ask the patient if he has any questions or concerns.
- Ensure that he is comfortable.
- Thank him.

[Note] The principal complications of NG tube insertion are aspiration and tissue trauma.

Urological history

Before starting

- Introduce yourself to the patient.
- Explain that you are going to ask him some questions to uncover the nature of his urological complaint, and ask for consent to do this.
- Ensure that he is comfortable.

The history

- Name, age, and occupation.

Presenting complaint and history of presenting complaint

- Ask about the main presenting complaint. Ask open questions.
- Elicit the patient's ideas, concerns, and expectations.
- Determine the time course of events and the severity of the problem.
- Ask specifically about:
  - pain: for any pain, ask about site, radiation, intensity, character, onset, duration, relieving and aggravating factors, and associated factors
  - fever
  - frequency
  - urgency
  - dysuria
  - haematuria
  - nocturia
  - hesitancy and terminal dribbling (if male)
  - poor stream
  - incontinence
  - back pain, leg weakness, weight loss, anorexia
  - vaginal/urethral discharge, genital sores
  - testicular masses, testicular pain
  - sexual dysfunction
  - sexual contacts

Past medical history

- Past urological problems.
- Ask specifically about UTI, renal colic, diabetes mellitus, hypertension, and gout.
- Current, past, and childhood illnesses.
- Surgery.

Drug history

- Prescribed medication.
- Over-the-counter medication.
- Recreational drugs.
- Allergies.

Family history

- Parents, siblings, and children. In particular, has anyone in the family had a similar problem?
- Ask specifically about bladder cancer.

Social history

- Employment.
- Housing.
- Travel.
- Alcohol consumption.
- Smoking.

After taking the history

- Ask the patient if there is anything he might add that you have forgotten to ask about.
- Thank the patient.
- State that you would carry out an abdominal and genital exam and order some key investigations.
- Summarise your findings and offer a differential diagnosis.

Most common conditions likely to appear in a urological history station	
Urinary tract infection	Prostatism
Urinary incontinence	Sexually transmitted disease

Male genitalia examination

Specifications: You may be asked to examine the male genitalia on a real patient or, more likely, on a pelvic mannequin.

Before starting

- Introduce yourself to the patient.
- Explain the examination and ask for his consent to carry it out.
- Ask for a chaperone.
- Ask him to lie on the couch and expose his groin area.
- Ensure that he is comfortable.

 Ensure the patient's comfort and dignity at all times.

The examination

General inspection

- From the end of the couch observe the patient's general appearance. The patient's age can give you an indication of the most likely pathology.
- In particular, note the distribution of facial, axillary, and pubic hair.
- Look for gynaecomastia.

Inspection and examination of the male genitalia

- Warm your hands.
- Ensure that the patient is not in pain.

Penis

- Inspect the penis for lesions and ulcers.
- Retract the foreskin and examine the *glans penis* and the external urethral meatus. Is there a discharge? Can a discharge be expressed?
  - If there is a discharge, indicate that you would swab it for microscopy and culture.

Scrotum

- Inspect the scrotum. Are the testicles present? Is their lie normal? If a testicle is absent, is it retracted or undescended? If you find a scar, the absent testicle may have been surgically removed.
- Fix upon the patient's face and palpate:
  - the testis
  - the epididymis
  - the *vas deferens*
- If you locate a mass, try to get above it. If you cannot, it is likely to be a hernia so test for a cough impulse (see *Station 23*).
- Next, transilluminate the mass using a pen torch. Is it a cyst or a solid mass? If it is a cyst, is it a hydrocoele or an epididymal cyst? If it is a solid mass, is it tender? Is it testicular or epididymal?

- If you suspect a varicocoele, a collection of varicosities in the pampiniform venous plexus, examine the patient in the standing position and test for a cough impulse. **Note that varicocoeles are invariably left-sided.**

Figure 26. Normal testis and appendages (1), hydrocoele (2), epididymal cyst (3), and varicocoele (4).

Examination of the lymphatics

- Palpate the inguinal nodes in the inguinal crease. Remember that only the penis and scrotum drain to the inguinal nodes, as the testicles drain to the para-aortic lymph nodes.

After the examination

- Cover up the patient.
- Thank the patient.
- Ensure that he is comfortable.
- Summarise your findings and offer a differential diagnosis.

Most common conditions likely to appear in an examination of the male genitalia station	
Hydrocoele	Direct inguinal hernia (see *Station 23*)
Epididymal cyst	Penile ulcer(s)
Varicocoele	

Male catheterisation

Specifications: A male anatomical model in lieu of a patient.

Before starting

- Introduce yourself to the patient.
- Explain the procedure and ask for his consent to carry it out.
- Position him flat on the couch with legs apart and groin exposed.

The equipment

On a clean trolley, gather:

- A catheterisation pack.
- Saline solution.
- Sterile gloves.
- A 10 ml pre-filled syringe containing 2% lignocaine gel.

- A 12–16 french Foley catheter.
- A catheter bag.
- A 10 ml syringe containing sterile water.
- Adhesive tape.

The procedure

- Check the expiry date of the catheter.
- Open the catheter pack aseptically, and pour saline solution into the receiver.
- If pre-filled syringes are not provided with the pack, draw up 10 ml sterile water and 10 ml lignocaine gel into separate syringes.
- Wash and dry your hands.
- Put on sterile gloves.
- Drape the patient.
- Place a collecting vessel in the patient's *entre-jambes*.
- With your non-dominant hand, hold the penis with a sterile swab.
- With your dominant hand, retract the foreskin and clean the area around the urethral meatus with saline-soaked swabs.
- Coat the end of the catheter with lignocaine gel and instil 10 ml of lignocaine gel into the urethra. Hold the urethral meatus closed.
- Indicate that the anaesthetic needs about 5 minutes to work.
- Hold the penis so that it is vertical.
- Holding the catheter by its sleeve, gently and progressively insert it into the urethra.
- Once a stream of urine is obtained, inject 10 ml of sterile water to inflate the catheter's balloon, continually ensuring that this does not cause the patient any pain.
- Gently retract the catheter until a resistance is felt.
- Attach the catheter bag.
- Reposition the foreskin.
- Tape the catheter to the thigh.

After the procedure

- Ensure that the patient is comfortable.
- Thank the patient.
- Discard any rubbish.
- Record the date and time of catheterisation, type and size of catheter used, volume of water used to inflate the balloon, and volume of urine in the catheter bag.

Examiner's questions

Indications for catheterisation
- Hygienic care of bedridden patients.
- Monitoring of urine output.
- Acute urinary retention.
- Chronic obstruction.
- Collection of a specimen of uncontaminated urine.
- Irrigation of the bladder.
- Imaging of the urinary tract.

Contraindications
- Pelvic trauma.
- Previous stricture.
- Previous failure to catheterise.
- Severe phimosis.

Complications
- Paraphimosis (from failure to reposition the foreskin).
- Urethral perforation and creation of false passages.
- Bleeding.
- Infection.
- Urethral strictures.

Female catheterisation

Specifications: A female anatomical model in lieu of a patient.

Before starting

- Introduce yourself to the patient.
- Explain the procedure and ask for her consent to carry it out.
- Ask her to undress from the waist down and place a sheet over her.

The equipment

On a clean trolley, gather:

- Two pairs of sterile gloves.
- A catheterisation pack.
- Saline solution.
- A 12–16 french Foley catheter.
- A 10 ml pre-filled syringe containing 2% lignocaine gel.
- A 10 ml syringe containing sterile water.
- A catheter bag.
- Adhesive tape.

The procedure

- Open the catheter pack aseptically and pour antiseptic solution into the receiver.
- If pre-filled syringes are not provided with the pack, draw up 10 ml sterile water and 10 ml lignocaine into separate syringes.
- Wash and dry your hands.
- Put on both pairs of gloves (practise this – it's not easy).
- Ask the patient to remove her sheet and lie flat on the couch, bringing her heels to her buttocks and then letting her knees flop out.
- Drape the patient.
- Place a collecting vessel in the patient's *entre-jambes*.
- Use your non-dominant hand to separate the labia minora.
- Clean the area around the urethral meatus with saline-soaked swabs.
- Coat the end of the catheter with lignocaine gel and instil 5 ml of lignocaine into the urethra.
- Indicate that the anaesthetic needs about 5 minutes to work.
- Discard the outer pair of gloves.
- Holding the catheter by its sleeve, gently and progressively insert it into the urethra.
- Once a stream of urine is obtained, inject 10 ml of sterile water to inflate the catheter's balloon, continually ensuring that this does not cause the patient any pain.
- Gently retract the catheter until a resistance is felt.
- Attach the catheter bag.
- Tape the catheter to the thigh.

Clinical Skills for OSCEs

Figure 27. Preparing to insert the catheter.

After the procedure

- Ensure that the patient is comfortable.
- Thank the patient.
- Discard any rubbish.
- Record the date and time of catheterisation, type and size of catheter used, volume of water used to inflate the balloon, and volume of urine in the catheter bag.

History of headaches

'I'm very brave generally', he went on in a low voice: 'only today I happen to have a headache'.

Lewis Carroll, *Through the Looking Glass*

Before starting

- Introduce yourself to the patient.
- Explain that you are going to ask him some questions to uncover the nature of his headaches, and ask for his consent to do this.
- Ensure that he is comfortable.

The history

- Name, age, and occupation.

Presenting complaint and history and presenting complaint

First use open questions to get the patient's history, and elicit his ideas, concerns, and expectations.

Then ask specifically about:

- **S**ite.
- **O**nset.
- **C**haracter.
- **R**adiation.
- **A**ssociated factors.
  - Nausea and vomiting.
  - Visual disturbances (aura, double vision, fortification spectra).
  - Photophobia.
  - Fever, chills.
  - Weight loss.
  - Rash.
  - Tender temporal arteries.
  - Neck pain, stiffness.
  - Myalgia.
  - Rhinorrhoea, lacrimation.
  - Altered level of consciousness.
  - Neurological deficit.
- **T**iming.
- **E**xacerbating and relieving factors (activity, caffeine, alcohol, dehydration, stress, eye strain, coughing/sneezing, bright lights, menses, hunger, certain foods).
- **S**everity (effect on the patient's life).

Socrates (470–399 BC)

Being asked whether it is better to marry or not, he (Socrates) replied, 'Whichever you do you will repent it.'

Diogenes (412–323BC), Ancient Greek Philosopher and founder of Cynicism

Past medical history

- Current, past, and childhood illnesses.
- Ask specifically about headache, migraine, intracranial lesions, and travel sickness as a child.
- Surgery.

Drug history

- Prescribed medication. Ask specifically about withdrawal from NSAIDs, opioids, glyceryl trinitrate, and calcium channel blockers.
- Over-the-counter medication.
- Recreational drugs.
- Allergies.

Social history

- Employment, past and present.
- Housing.
- Mood. Depression is a common cause of headaches.
- Smoking.
- Alcohol use. Alcohol is a common cause of headaches.

Family history

- Parents, siblings, and children.
- Ask about migraine and travel sickness.

After taking the history

- Ask the patient if there is anything he might like to add that you have forgotten to ask about.
- Ask him if he has any questions or concerns.
- Thank him.
- Summarise your findings and offer a differential diagnosis.
- State that you would like to carry out a physical examination and some investigations to confirm your diagnosis and exclude life-threatening causes of headaches (see box below).

Most common conditions likely to appear in a headaches history station	
Tension headaches	Cervical spondylosis
Cluster headaches	Intracranial mass lesions, e.g. tumour
Migraines	Meningitis
Cranial arteritis	Subarachnoid haemorrhage

History of 'funny turns'

Before starting

- Introduce yourself to the patient.
- Explain that you are going to ask him some questions to uncover the cause of his collapse, and ask for his consent to do this.
- Ensure that he is comfortable.

The history

- Name, age, and occupation.

Presenting complaint and history of presenting complaint

First use open questions to get the patient's story, and elicit their ideas, concerns and expectations.

Think about the common causes of a funny turn, as these should inform your line of questioning.

Most common conditions likely to appear in a history of 'funny turns' station	
Syncope (simple faint)	Postural hypotension (drugs, dehydration, autonomic dysfunction …)
Seizure/pseudoseizure	Carotid sinus syndrome
Transient ischaemic attack	Hypoglycaemia
Arrhythmia	Vertebrobasilar insufficiency

Ask about:

- If the patient remembers falling.
- The circumstances of the fall:
  - had the patient just arisen from bed? (postural hypotension)
  - did the patient suffer an intense emotion? (syncope)
  - had the patient been coughing or straining? (syncope)
  - had the patient been extending his neck? (vertebrobasilar insufficiency)
  - did the patient have any palpitations? (arrhythmia)
- Any loss of consciousness and its duration.
- Prodromal symptoms such as aura, change in mood, strange feeling in the gut, sensation of déjà vu.
- Fitting, frothing at the mouth, tongue biting, incontinence.
- Headache or confusion upon recovery.
- Injuries sustained.
- Previous episodes.

Past medical history

- Current, past, and childhood illnesses. Ask specifically about epilepsy, heart problems, stroke, diabetes (autonomic neuropathy), cervical spondylosis, and arthritis.
- Surgery.

Drug history

- Prescribed medication. Drugs such as antipsychotics, tricyclic antidepressants, and antihypertensives can cause postural hypotension. Insulin can cause hypoglycaemia.
- Over-the-counter medication.
- Recreational drugs.
- Recent changes in medication.

Family history

- Parents, siblings, and children.
- Ask specifically about epilepsy and heart problems.

Social history

- Smoking.
- Alcohol use.
- Employment, past and present.
- Housing.
- Effect of falls on patient's life.

After taking the history

- Ask the patient if there is anything he might add that you have forgotten to ask about.
- Ask him if he has any questions or concerns.
- Thank him.
- Summarise your findings and offer a differential diagnosis.
- State that you would like to carry out a physical examination and some investigations to confirm your diagnosis.

Cranial nerve examination

Specifications: You may be asked to limit your examination to certain cranial nerves only, e.g. I–VI, VII–XII.

Before starting

- Introduce yourself to the patient.
- Explain the examination and ask for his consent to carry it out.
- Ensure that he is comfortable.

The examination

The olfactory nerve (CN I)

- Ask the patient if he has noticed a change in his sense of smell or taste. If he has, indicate that you would perform an olfactory examination by asking the patient to smell different scents, e.g. mint or coffee.

The optic nerve (CN II)

(See *Station 47: Vision and the eye examination* for more details.)

- Test visual acuity on a Snellen chart.
- Test near vision by asking the patient to read test types (or a page in a book).
- Indicate that you could use Ishihara plates to test colour vision.
- Test the visual fields by confrontation.
- Examine the eyes by direct fundoscopy.

The oculomotor, trochlear, and abducens nerves (CN III, IV, and VI)

(See *Station 47: Vision and the eye examination* for more details.)

- Inspect the eyes, paying particular attention to the size and symmetry of the pupils, and excluding a visible ptosis (Horner's syndrome) or squint.
- Test the direct and consensual pupillary light reflexes. Explain that you are going to shine a bright light into the patient's eye and that this may feel uncomfortable.
- Perform the cover test. Ask the patient to fixate on a point and cover one eye. Observe the movement of the uncovered eye. Repeat the test for the other eye.
- Examine eye movements. Ask the patient to keep his head still and to follow your finger with his eyes, and to tell you if he sees double at any point. Look out for nystagmus at the extremes of gaze.
- Test the accommodation reflex. Ask the patient to follow your finger in to his nose.

Clinical Skills for OSCEs

Figure 28. Horner's syndrome. Characteristic features are ipsilateral ptosis, miosis, apparent enophthalmos, and anhydrosis and vasodilatation on the same side of the face.

Reproduced from Otolaryngology – Houston at www.ghorayeb.com with permission.

The trigeminal nerve (CN V)

Sensory part

- Test light touch in the three branches of the trigeminal nerve. Compare both sides.
- Indicate that you could test the corneal reflex, but that this is likely to cause the patient some discomfort.

Figure 29. The three branches of the trigeminal nerve. 'Trigeminal' means 'three twins'.

Motor part

- Test the muscles of mastication (the temporalis, masseter, and pterygoid muscles) by asking the patient to:
  - clench his teeth (palpate his temporalis and masseter muscles bilaterally)
  - open and close his mouth against resistance (place your fist under his chin)
- Indicate that you could test the jaw jerk. Ask the patient to let his mouth fall open slightly. Place your fingers on his chin and tap them lightly with a tendon hammer.

The facial nerve (CN VII)

- Look for facial asymmetry. Note that the nasolabial folds and the angle of the mouth are especially indicative of facial asymmetry.

Sensory part

- Indicate that you could test the anterior two-thirds of the tongue for sensation.

Motor part

- Test the muscles of facial expression by asking the patient to:
  - lift his eyebrows as far as they will go
  - close his eyes as tightly as possible (try to open them)
  - blow out his cheeks
  - purse his lips or whistle
  - show his teeth

The acoustic nerve (CN VIII)

(See *Station 46: Hearing and the ear examination* for more details.)

- Test hearing sensitivity in each ear by occluding one ear and rubbing your thumb and fingers together in front of the other. Pretend that you are in private practice and asking for your fee.
- Indicate that you could carry out the Rinne and Weber tests and examine the ears by auroscopy (see *Station 46*).

The glossopharyngeal nerve (CN IX)

- Indicate that you could test the gag reflex by touching the tonsillar fossae on both sides, but that this is likely to cause the patient some discomfort.

The vagus nerve (CN X)

- Ask the patient to phonate (say 'aaah') and, aided by a pen torch, look for deviation of the uvula.

The hypoglossal nerve (CN XII)

- Aided by a pen torch, inspect the tongue for wasting and fasciculation.
- Ask the patient to stick out his tongue and to wiggle it from side to side.

The accessory nerve (CN XI)

- Look for wasting of the sternocleidomastoid and trapezius muscles.

- Ask the patient to:
  - shrug his shoulders against resistance
  - turn his head to either side against resistance

After the examination

- Thank the patient.
- Ensure that he is comfortable.
- If appropriate, state that you would order some key investigations, e.g. a CT or MRI.
- Summarise your findings and offer a differential diagnosis.

Most common conditions likely to appear or to be asked about in a cranial nerves examination station	
Third nerve palsy	Pseudo-bulbar palsy
Bell's palsy	Brain-stem infarction
Horner's syndrome	Multiple sclerosis
Cavernous sinus lesions	Motor neurone disease
Cerebellopontine angle tumour	Myasthenia gravis
Bulbar palsy	

Motor system of the upper limbs examination

Before starting

- Introduce yourself to the patient.
- Explain the examination and ask for his permission to carry it out.
- Position him and ask him to expose his arms.
- Ask if he is currently experiencing any pain.

The examination

Inspection

- Look for abnormal posturing.
- Look for abnormal movements such as tremor, fasciculation, dystonia, athetosis.
- Assess the muscles of the hands, arms, and shoulder girdle for size, shape, and symmetry. You can also measure the circumference of the arms.

Tone

- Ensure that the patient is not in any pain.
- Test the tone in the upper limbs by holding the patient's hand and simultaneously pronating and supinating and flexing and extending the forearm. If you suspect increased tone, ask the patient to clench his teeth and re-test. Is the increased tone best described as spasticity (clasp-knife) or as rigidity (lead pipe)? Spasticity suggests a pyramidal lesion, rigidity suggests an extra-pyramidal lesion.

Power

- Test muscle strength for shoulder abduction, elbow flexion and extension, wrist flexion and extension, finger flexion, extension, abduction and adduction, and thumb abduction and op-position. Compare muscle strength on both sides, and grade it on the MRC muscle strength scale:
  - **0** No movement.
  - **1** Feeble contractions.
  - **2** Movement, but not against gravity.
  - **3** Movement against gravity, but not against resistance.
  - **4** Movement against resistance, but not to full strength.
  - **5** Full strength.

Table 12. Important root values in the upper limb – muscle strength	
Shoulder abduction	C5
Elbow flexion	C6
Elbow extension	C7
Wrist extension	C6, C7
Wrist flexion	C7, C8
Finger extension	C7 (radial nerve)
Finger flexion	C8
Finger abduction/adduction	T1 (ulnar nerve)
Thumb abduction/opposition	T1 (median nerve)

Reflexes

- Test biceps, supinator, and triceps reflexes with a tendon hammer. Compare both sides. If a reflex cannot be elicited, ask the patient to clench his teeth and re-test (reinforcement).

Table 13. Important root values in the upper limb – reflexes	
Biceps	C5, C6
Supinator	C6
Triceps	C7

Cerebellar signs

- Test for intention tremor, dysynergia, and dysmetria by asking the patient to carry out the finger-to-nose test.
  - Place your index finger at about 2 feet from the patient's face. Ask him to touch the tip of his nose and then the tip of your finger with the tip of his index finger. Once he is able to do this, ask him to do it as fast as he can. And remember that he has two hands!
- Then test for dysdiadochokinesis.
  - Ask the patient to clap and then show him how to clap by alternating the palmar and dorsal surfaces of one hand. Once he is able to do this, ask him to do it as fast as he can. Ask him to repeat the test with his other hand.

After the examination

- Thank the patient.
- Ensure that he is comfortable.
- Ask to carry out a full neurological examination.
- If appropriate, indicate that you would order some key investigations, e.g. CT, MRI, nerve conduction studies, electromyography, etc.
- Summarise your findings and offer a differential diagnosis.

Most common conditions likely to appear in an upper limbs motor examination station	
Parkinson's disease	Radiculopathy
Cerebellar syndrome	Myopathy
Ulnar, median, or radial nerve lesion	Hemiplegia

Sensory system of the upper limbs examination

Before starting

- Introduce yourself to the patient.
- Explain the examination and ask for his permission to carry it out.
- Position him so that he is comfortably seated and ask him to expose his arms.
- Ask if he is currently experiencing any pain.

The examination

To examine the sensory system, test light touch, pain, vibration sense, and proprioception.

 Do not forget to inspect the arms before you start.

- Light touch (not light rub). Ask the patient to close his eyes and apply a wisp of cotton wool to the sternum and then to each of the dermatomes of the arm. Do not forget to compare both sides as you go along.

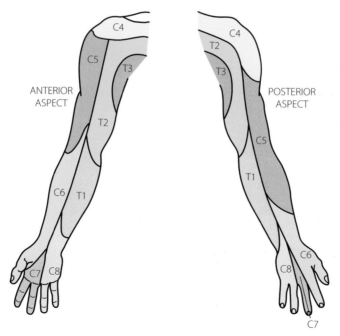

Figure 30. Dermatomes of the arm.

- Pain. Ask the patient to close his eyes and apply a sharp object – ideally a neurological pin – to the sternum and then to each of the dermatomes of the arm. Compare both sides as you go along.
- Vibration. Ask the patient to close his eyes and apply a vibrating 128 Hz or 256 Hz tuning fork (not the smaller 512 Hz tuning fork used in hearing tests) to the sternum and then over the bony prominences of the upper arm. Compare both sides as you go along.
- Proprioception. Ask the patient to close his eyes. Hold one of his fingers by its sides and move it at the distal interphalangeal joint, asking him to identify the direction of each movement. Before you do this, ensure that the patient does not suffer from arthritis or from some other painful condition of the hand.

After the examination

- Thank the patient.
- Ensure that he is comfortable.
- Ask to carry out a full neurological examination.
- Summarise your findings and offer a differential diagnosis.

Most common conditions likely to appear in an upper limbs sensory examination station
Radiculopathy, affecting a single nerve root, e.g. C6
Mononeuropathy, affecting a single nerve, e.g. ulnar nerve
Polyneuropathy, affecting multiple nerves as in diabetic neuropathy
Cortical lesions, e.g. Brown–Séquard syndrome

Motor system of the lower limbs examination

Before starting

- Introduce yourself to the patient.
- Explain the examination and ask for his permission to carry it out.
- Position him and ask him to expose his legs.
- Ask if he is currently experiencing any pain.

The examination

Inspection

- Look for deformities of the foot.
- Look for abnormal posturing.
- Look for fasciculation.
- Assess the muscles of the legs for size, shape, and symmetry. You can also measure the circumference of the quadriceps or calves.

Tone

- Ensure that the patient is not in any pain.
- Test the tone in the legs by rolling the leg on the bed, by flexing and extending the knee, or by abruptly lifting the leg at the knee.

Power

- Test muscle strength for hip flexion, extension, abduction and adduction, knee flexion and extension, plantar flexion and dorsiflexion of the foot and big toe, and inversion and eversion of the forefoot. Compare muscle strength on both sides, and grade it on the MRC scale for muscle strength:
  0 No movement.
  1 Feeble contractions.
  2 Movement, but not against gravity.
  3 Movement against gravity, but not against resistance.
  4 Movement against resistance, but not to full strength.
  5 Full strength.

Table 14. Important root values in the lower limb – muscle strength	
Hip flexion	L1, L2
Hip extension	S1
Hip adduction	L2
Knee flexion	L5, S1
Knee extension	L3, L4
Foot dorsiflexion	L4, L5
Foot plantar flexion	S1
Big toe dorsiflexion	L5

Reflexes

- Test the knee jerk and ankle jerk with a tendon hammer. Compare both sides. If a reflex cannot be elicited, ask the patient to clench his teeth and re-test (reinforcement).

Table 15. Important root values in the lower limb – reflexes	
Knee jerk	L3, L4
Ankle jerk	S1

- Test for clonus by holding up the ankle and rapidly dorsiflexing the foot.
- Test for the Babinsky sign (extensor plantar reflex) using the sharp end of a tendon hammer or an orange stick. The sign is positive if there is extension of the big toe at the MTP joint, so-called 'upgoing plantars'.

Cerebellar signs

- Carry out the heel-to-shin test.
  - Lie the patient on a couch. Ask him to run the heel of one leg down the shin of the other, and then to bring the heel back up to the knee and to start again. Ask him to repeat the test with his other leg.

Gait

- If he can, ask the patient to walk to the end of the room and to turn around and walk back. (See *Station 36: Gait, co-ordination, and cerebellar function examination*.)

Figure 31. Testing for the Babinsky or extensor plantar sign.

After the examination

- Thank the patient.
- Ensure that he is comfortable.
- Ask to carry out a full neurological examination.
- If appropriate, indicate that you would order some key investigations, e.g. CT, MRI, nerve conduction studies, electromyography, etc.
- Summarise your findings and offer a differential diagnosis.

Most common conditions likely to appear in a lower limbs motor examination station	
Radiculopathy	Hemiplegia
Polyneuropathy	Myopathy
Cauda equina lesion	Foot drop

Station 35

Sensory system of the lower limbs examination

Before starting

- Introduce yourself to the patient.
- Explain the examination and ask for his permission to carry it out.
- Position him on a couch and ask him to expose his legs.
- Ask if he is currently experiencing any pain.

The examination

To examine the sensory system, test light touch, pain, vibration sense, and proprioception.

 Do not forget to inspect the legs before you start.

- Light touch (*not* light rub): ask the patient to close his eyes and apply a wisp of cotton wool to the sternum and then to each of the dermatomes of the leg. Do not forget to compare both sides as you go along.

Figure 32. Dermatomes of the leg.

- Pain. Ask the patient to close his eyes and apply a sharp object – ideally a neurological pin – to the sternum and then to each of the dermatomes of the leg. Compare both sides as you go along.
- Vibration. Ask the patient to close his eyes and apply a vibrating 128 Hz or 256 Hz tuning fork (not the smaller 512 Hz tuning fork used in hearing tests) to the sternum and then over the bony prominences of the leg. Compare both sides as you go along.
- Proprioception. Ask the patient to close his eyes. Hold one of his toes by its sides and move it at the interphalangeal joint, asking him to identify the direction of each movement. Before you do this, ensure that the patient does not suffer from arthritis, gout, or some other painful condition of the foot. If the patient is able to stand, you can also perform Romberg's test (see *Station 36: Gait, co-ordination, and cerebellar function examination.*)

After the examination

- Thank the patient.
- Ensure that he is comfortable.
- Ask to carry out a full neurological examination.
- If appropriate, indicate that you would order some key investigations, e.g. CT, MRI, nerve conduction studies, electromyography, etc.
- Summarise your findings and offer a differential diagnosis.

Most common conditions likely to appear in a lower limbs sensory examination station	
Radiculopathy	*Cauda equina* lesion
Mononeuropathy	Cortical lesion
Polyneuropathy	

Station 36

Gait, co-ordination, and cerebellar function examination

Before starting

- Introduce yourself to the patient.
- Explain the examination and ask for his consent to carry it out.
- Ask if he is currently experiencing any pain.

Examination of gait

- Inspection. Ask the patient to stand up. Ensure that he is steady on his feet and inspect his posture from both front and side. Truncal ataxia suggests a midline cerebellar lesion.
- Gait and arm swing. Ask him to walk to the end of the room and to turn around and walk back. If he normally uses a stick or frame, he should not be prevented from doing so.
- Heel-to-toe test. Ask him to walk heel-to-toe, 'as if on a tightrope'. Ataxia on a narrow-based gait suggests a cerebellar or vestibular lesion.
- Romberg's test. Ask him to stand unaided with his arms by his sides and with his eyes closed. If he sways and threatens to lose his balance, the test is said to be positive, indicating posterior column disease.

 You must be in a position to steady the patient should he threaten to fall.

Table 16. Abnormal gaits	
Hemiplegic gait	The pelvis tilts upwards, the hip is abducted, and the leg is swung forwards in a semi-circular movement. The leg is stiff and extended but the arm may be held in flexion and adduction with minimal swing.
Scissor gait	A spastic gait seen in cerebral palsy and resulting from muscle contractures. The hips, knees, and ankles are flexed, producing a crouching and tiptoeing appearance. In addition, the hips are adducted and internally rotated, such that the knees cross or hit each other in a scissor-like movement.
Festinating gait	Seen in Parkinson's disease. Short shuffling steps with stiff arms and legs and stooped posture. Difficulty starting and turning.
Ataxic gait	Seen in spinal and cerebellar lesions and in alcohol intoxication. Unsteady, broad-based gait with a lurching quality.
Neuropathic gait	Seen in peripheral neuropathies. Weak foot dorsiflexors result in a high-stepping gait with foot-slapping. The high-stepping is an attempt to prevent the foot from dragging and being injured. Also called 'high-stepping gait' or 'foot-slapping gait'.
Trendelenburg gait	Seen in weakness of the hip abductors or in an inability or reluctance to abduct the hip, e.g. due to a fractured neck of femur or to arthritic pain. The pelvis tilts to the unaffected side in the stance phase. As a result, the trunk lurches to the affected side in an attempt to maintain a level pelvis. Bilateral Trendelenburg results in a typical waddling gait.
Antalgic gait	Seen in arthritis and trauma. Avoidance of motions that trigger pain. Often quick, short, and light footsteps. Not to be confused with a Trendelenburg gait.
Myopathic gait	In muscular diseases the proximal pelvic girdle muscles are most affected, such that the patient is unable to stabilise the pelvis in the stance phase. The pelvis drops to the side of the leg being raised, and this results in a broad-based, waddling gait.

Examination of co-ordination

- Resting tremor. Ask the patient to rest his hands in his lap and to close his eyes. Resting tremor is a sign of Parkinson's disease.
- Intention tremor. Ask the patient to do something, e.g. remove his watch or write a sentence.
- Examine muscle tone in the elbow (flexion and extension) and wrist (flexion and extension, abduction and adduction) joints. Compare both sides.
- Dysdiadochokinesis. Ask the patient to clap and then show him how to clap by alternating the palmar and dorsal surfaces of one hand. Once he is able to do this, ask him to do it as fast as he can. Ask him to repeat the test with his other hand.
- Finger-to-nose test. Place your index finger at about 2 feet from the patient's face. Ask him to touch the tip of his nose and then the tip of your finger with the tip of his index finger. Once he is able to do this, ask him to do it as fast as he can. And remember that he has two hands! Look for intention tremor and dysmetria (past-pointing), both signs of cerebellar disease.
- Fine finger movements. Ask the patient to oppose his thumb with each of his other fingers in turn. Once he is able to do this, ask him to do it as fast as he can. Again, remember that he has two hands.
- Heel-to-shin test. Lie the patient on a couch. Ask him to run the heel of one leg down the shin of the other, and then to bring the heel back up to the knee and to start again. Ask him to repeat the test with his other leg.

Assessment of cerebellar function

- If you are specifically asked to assess cerebellar function, carry out the above plus test eye movements (nystagmus) and ask the patient to say 'baby hippopotamus' (slurred/ staccato speech). If you are then asked to list cerebellar signs, simply remember the acronym DANISH:
  - **D**ysdiadochokinesis and dysmetria (finger overshoot)
  - **A**taxia
  - **N**ystagmus – test eye movements
  - **I**ntention tremor
  - **S**lurred/staccato speech – ask the patient to say 'baby hippopotamus' or 'British constitu- tion'
  - **H**ypotonia/hyporeflexia

After the examination

- Ask the patient if he has any questions or concerns.
- Thank the patient.
- Ensure that he is comfortable.
- Summarise your findings and offer a differential diagnosis.

Most common conditions likely to appear in a gait and co-ordination station	
Hemiplegia	Peripheral neuropathy
Parkinson's disease	Severe arthritis
Cerebellar ataxia	Musculoskeletal disease

Station 37

Speech assessment

The patient is likely to find the assessment difficult and distressing, so remember to be especially empathetic. In particular, do not rush the examination or keep on interrupting the patient, but move at a pace that feels comfortable for him.

Table 17. Definitions	
Dysphonia	Impairment of ability to vocalise speech.
Dysarthria	Impairment of ability to articulate speech.
Dysphasia	Impairment of ability to comprehend or express language.
Expressive dysphasia (Broca's area, in the inferolateral dominant frontal lobe) and receptive dysphasia (Wernicke's area, in the posterior superior dominant temporal lobe) often co-exist.	

Before starting

- Introduce yourself to the patient.
- Explain the assessment and obtain his consent to carry it out.
- Ask him to try to describe his current problems.

The assessment

Orientation in time and place

Time

Name: (year) (season) (month) (date) (day)

Place

Name: (country) (county/region) (town) (hospital) (floor)

Dysphasia

Expressive

Assess whether the patient has difficulty in finding the right words whilst in conversation with you.

Nominal

Ask the patient to name some common objects such as a watch, pen, or penny coin; then to name the components of some of these objects, e.g. hour hand, winder, strap. Note that nominal dysphasia is a common form of expressive dysphasia.

Receptive

Assess whether the patient has difficulty understanding you by asking him to carry out some simple instructions such as 'shut your eyes', 'touch your nose', and 'point to the door'.

Dysarthria

Ask the patient to repeat some of the following: 'British constitution', 'West Register Street', 'Baby hippopotamus', 'Biblical criticism', and 'Artillery'.

Assess the structures involved in phonation and articulation by asking the patient to repeat:

- 'Me, me, me'   Lips
- 'La, la, la'   Tongue
- 'Khu, gut'   Palate
- 'Ah'   Palate, larynx, and expiratory muscles

Dysphonia

- Make a note of the patient's volume of speech, which may be low if there is weakness of the vocal cords or respiratory muscles.

Dyslexia

- Correct the patient's vision and ask him to read a short paragraph from a newspaper or magazine, and bear in mind that not all people who can't read are dyslexic!

Dysgraphia

- Ask the patient to write a sentence.

After the assessment

- Ask the patient if he has any questions or concerns.
- Thank the patient.
- Summarise your findings, offer a differential diagnosis, and state the probable area of the lesion.

Most common conditions likely to appear in a speech assessment station	
Stroke	Parkinson's disease
Dementia	Myasthenia gravis
Depressive disorder	

General psychiatric history

Specifications: The instructions for this station are likely to ask you to focus on one part of the history, e.g. presenting complaint and history of presenting complaint, social history, personal history.

 In taking a psychiatric history, it is especially important to put the patient at ease and to be seen to be sensitive, tactful, and empathetic.

Before starting

- Introduce yourself to the patient.
- Ensure that he is comfortable. Make some general comments to put him at ease and build a rapport.

The history

- Name, age, and mode of referral (if not already provided).

Presenting complaint and history of presenting complaint

- Ask mainly open questions, e.g. *Can you tell me why you've come to the hospital today?* Try to form a diagnostic hypothesis and to validate or falsify it by asking further questions (logico-deductive approach).
- Ask about:
  - the onset and duration of symptoms
  - the effect the symptoms are having on the patient's everyday life
  - any treatments so far
- If you have not done so already, ask screening questions about mood, anxiety, obsessions, abnormal beliefs, and abnormal perceptions (see *Station 39: Mental state examination*).

Informant history

If the patient is accompanied by a relative, friend, or carer, an informant history should be taken at this stage.

Past psychiatric history

- Previous episodes of illness.
- Previous treatments and their outcomes.
- Previous admissions, formal and informal.
- History of neglect or self-harm.
- History of violence.

Past medical history

- Current illness:
  - acute illness
  - chronic illness
  - vascular risk factors

- Past and childhood illnesses, including head injury.
- Surgery.

Drug history/current treatments

- Psychological treatments.
- Prescribed medication.
- Recent changes in prescribed medication.
- Over-the-counter drugs.
- Allergies.

Substance use

- Alcohol.
- Tobacco.
- Illicit drugs.

[Note] Further questioning to establish dependence may be required if alcohol use and/or illicit drug use is high (see *Station 43: Alcohol history*).

Family history

- Determine if anyone in the family has suffered from psychiatric illness or attempted suicide, e.g. *"Has anyone in the family ever had a nervous breakdown?"*
- Partner: age or age at death, occupation, health.
- Children: age or age at death, occupation, health.
- Quality of relationships and atmosphere in the home.
- Recent events in the family.

Social history

- Self-care.
- Social support.
- Housing.
- Finances.
- Typical day.
- Interests and hobbies.
- Predominant mood and premorbid personality.

Personal history

- Birth.
- Developmental milestones.
- Childhood: emotional problems, serious illnesses, prolonged separation from parents.
- Educational achievement.
- Occupational history.
- Forensic history.
- Psychosexual history: past and present partners (including same sex partners), quality of relationships, frequency of sexual intercourse, sexual problems, physical or sexual abuse.
- Forensic history, e.g. *"Have you ever had problems with the police or with the law?"*
- Religious or spiritual orientation, e.g. *"Do you believe there is something beyond us, like God?"*

After taking the history

- Ask the patient if there is anything he might add that you have forgotten to ask about.
- Summarise your findings and offer a differential diagnosis.
- Thank the patient.

Most common conditions likely to appear in a psychiatric history station
Depressive disorder
Anxiety disorder, e.g. agoraphobia, social phobia, panic disorder, generalised anxiety disorder
Mixed depression—anxiety
Obsessive—compulsive disorder
Eating disorder
Mania and bipolar affective disorder
Schizophrenia and other delusional disorders

Mental state examination

Specifications: The instructions for this station are likely to ask you to focus on one part of the mental state examination only, or to omit cognitive assessment. In some places, the patient-actor might by replaced by a real patient on a video recording.

Before starting

- Introduce yourself to the patient.
- Explain that you would like to explore his thoughts and feelings, and ask him if this is OK.
- Take out a pen and pad!

Assessing the mental state

The mental state can be assessed under 7 main headings:
1. Appearance and behaviour.
2. Speech.
3. Mood.
4. Abnormal thoughts.
5. Abnormal experiences.
6. Cognition.
7. Insight.

Appearance and behaviour

Begin by asking the patient some open questions, and focusing your attention on his *appearance and behaviour*.

- Level of consciousness.
- Appearance: body build, posture, general physical condition, grooming and hygiene, dress, physical stigmata such as scars, piercings, and tattoos.
- Inappropriate behaviour and attitude to the examiner. In particular note: facial expression, degree of eye contact, and quality of rapport.
- Motor activity/disorders of movement, e.g. agitation, retardation, tremor, dystonias, mannerisms.

Speech

Note:

- Amount, rate, volume, and tone of speech, e.g. logorrhoea, pressure of speech, poverty of speech, mutism.
- Form of speech, e.g. tangentiality, circumstantiality, clang associations, neologisms, perseverations.

Mood

Note or ask about:

- Affect.
- Current mood state and severity. If there is the suggestion of a mood disorder, this should be explored further (see *Station 41: Depression history*).
- Biological symptoms: sleep, appetite, libido, energy.
- Ideas of harm to self, e.g. *"People with problems similar to those that you have been describing often feel that life is no longer worth living. Have you felt that life is no longer worth living? (Yes) Have you actually thought of killing yourself?"*
- Ideas of harm to others.
- Anxiety and anxiety symptoms, e.g. butterflies, giddiness, clamminess, palpitations, difficulty catching breath. If there is the suggestion of an anxiety disorder, this should be explored further.

 You are likely to fail this station if you do not ask about ideas of harm in an at-risk patient.

Abnormal thoughts

Note or ask about:

- Stream of thought, e.g. pressure of thought, poverty of thought, thought blocking.
- Form of thought, e.g. flight of ideas, loosening of associations, over-inclusive thinking.
- Content of thought.
  - Preoccupations, ruminations, obsessions, and compulsive acts, e.g. for obsessions, *"Do certain things keep coming into your mind even though you try hard to keep them out?"* And for compulsive acts, *"Do you ever find yourself spending a lot of time doing the same thing over and over again even though you've already done it well enough?"*
  - Phobias, e.g. *"Do you have any special fears, like some people are afraid of spiders or snakes?"*
  - Delusions and overvalued ideas. For obvious reasons, you cannot easily ask directly about delusions. Begin by an introductory statement and general questions, such as *"I would like to ask you some questions that might seem a little bit strange. These are questions that we ask to everyone who comes to see us. Is that all right with you? Do you have any ideas that your friends and family do not share?"* Explore any delusions and in particular ask about their onset, their effect on the patient's life, and the patient's explanation for them (degree of insight). If necessary, ask specifically about common delusional themes, e.g. delusions of persecution, reference, and control.

Abnormal experiences

Ask about:

- Illusions and hallucinations. Again begin by an introductory statement and general questions, such as *"I gather that you have been under quite some pressure recently. When people are under pressure they sometimes find that their imagination plays tricks on them. Have you had any such experiences? Have you seen things which other people cannot see? Have you heard things which other people cannot hear?"* Ask about all five modalities and explore any positive findings for content, onset, frequency, duration, and effect on the patient's life. Exclude pseudohallucinations and hypnogogic and hypnopompic hallucinations. For auditory hallucinations of voices, determine if there is more than one voice, and if the voices talk to the patient (second person) or about him (third person). If the voices talk to him, do they command him to do dangerous things and, importantly, is he likely to act on these commands? If the voices talk about him, do they comment on his every thought and action (running commentary)? Other forms of auditory hallucinations are *écho de la pensée* and *gedankenlautwerden*, both first rank symptoms of schizophrenia.

• Depersonalisation and derealisation, e.g. for depersonalisation *'Have you ever felt unreal?'* And for derealisation, *'Have you ever felt that things around you are unreal?'*

Cognition

See *Station 40: Cognitive assessment – the Folstein Mini-Mental State Examination.*

Insight

To determine degree of insight, ask the patient:

• *"Do you think there is anything wrong with you?"*

If no,

• *"Why did you come to hospital?"*

If yes,

• *"What do you think is wrong with you?"*
• *"What do you think the cause of it is?"*
• *"Do you think you need treatment?"*
• *"What are you hoping treatment will do for you?"*

After the mental state examination

• Thank the patient.
• Ensure that he is comfortable.
• Summarise your findings. Note that mood should be reported as subjective mood and objective mood. Do not omit to comment upon risk.
• Offer a differential diagnosis.

Table 18. Principal features of key psychiatric disorders See ICD-10 or DSM-IV for detailed diagnostic criteria.	
Depressive disorder	See *Station 41*
Mania	• Garish clothing, accessories, and makeup
	• Hyperactive, flirtatious, hypervigilant, assertive, and/or aggressive behaviour
	• Pressured speech; abnormalities of the form of speech
	• Euphoric or irritable or labile mood
	• Grandiose thoughts with flight of ideas and loosening of associations; mood congruent delusions
	• Hallucinations
	• Poor concentration
	• Poor insight
Schizophrenia	• Delusions
	• Hallucinations
	• Disorganised speech
	• Disorganised or catatonic behaviour
	• Negative symptoms

continued

Table 18. Principal features of key psychiatric disorders – *continued*

Agoraphobia	Persistent irrational fear of places difficult or embarrassing to escape from, such as places that are confined, crowded, or far from home. Increased reliance on trusted companions for accompaniment or, in severe cases, restriction to the home.
Social phobia	Persistent irrational fear of being scrutinised by others and of being embarrassed or humiliated, either in most social situations or in specific social situations such as public speaking.
Specific phobia	Persistent irrational fear of one or more objects or situations. Common specific phobias include heights, darkness, enclosed spaces, storms, animals, flying, driving, blood, injections, and dental and medical procedures.
Panic disorder	Panic attacks are characterised by rapid onset of severe anxiety lasting for about 20–30 minutes. They may occur in the phobic anxiety disorder listed above or in other disorders such as OCD, PTSD, and organic disorders.
	In panic disorder, panic attacks occur recurrently and unexpectedly. There is fear of the implications and consequences of an attack, e.g. having a heart attack, losing control, 'going crazy'. Anticipatory fear of panic attacks develops and may itself lead to further panic attacks and to significant behavioural changes such as the development of agoraphobia.
Generalised anxiety disorder	Long-standing free-floating anxiety that may fluctuate but that is neither situational (phobic anxiety disorders) nor episodic (panic disorder). There is apprehension about a number of events far out of proportion to the actual likelihood or impact of the feared events. Other common symptoms include symptoms of autonomic arousal, irritability, poor concentration, muscle tension, tiredness, and sleep disturbances.
Obsessive compulsive disorder (OCD)	An obsessional thought is a recurrent idea, image, or impulse that is perceived as being senseless, that is unsuccessfully resisted, and that results in marked anxiety and distress.
	A compulsive act is a recurrent stereotyped behaviour that is not useful or enjoyable but that reduces anxiety and distress. It is usually perceived as being senseless and is unsuccessfully resisted. A compulsive act may be a response to an obsessive thought or according to rules that must be applied rigidly.
Post-traumatic stress disorder (PTSD)	A protracted and sometimes delayed response to a highly threatening or catastrophic experience characterised by numbing, detachment, flashbacks, nightmares, partial or complete amnesia for the event, avoidance of (and distress at) reminders of the event, and prominent anxiety symptoms. Associated psychiatric disorders are very common, especially depressive disorders, anxiety disorders, and alcohol and substance misuse.
Adjustment disorder	A protracted response to a significant life change or life event characterised by depressive symptoms and/or anxiety symptoms that are not severe enough to meet a diagnosis of depressive disorder or anxiety disorder, but that nevertheless lead to an impairment of social functioning.
Somatisation disorder (Briquet's syndrome)	A long history of multiple and severe physical symptoms that cannot be accounted for by a physical disorder or other psychiatric disorder. Compare to factitious disorders such as Münchausen syndrome and to malingering.
Hypochondriacal disorder (hypochondriasis)	A fear or belief of having a serious physical disorder despite medical reassurance to the contrary.
Eating disorders	See *Station 44*.
Alcohol dependence	See *Station 43*.

Cognitive assessment – the Folstein Mini-Mental State Examination (MMSE)

Generally speaking, a quick and informal cognitive assessment can be carried out by recording the following:

- Orientation in time, place, and person
- Attention and concentration, e.g. serial sevens test. Record the time taken and the number of errors
- Memory:
  - short-term memory
  - recent memory
  - remote memory
- Grasp, e.g. name the prime minister and reigning monarch

If cognitive impairment is suspected, you can carry out the Folstein Mini-Mental State Examination (MMSE). The MMSE is scored out of 30. Scores of less than 22 are indicative of significant cognitive impairment, while scores of 22 to 25 are indicative of moderate cognitive impairment. The result is invalid if the patient is delirious or has an affective disorder. Due to recent copyright restrictions only some of the items on the MMSE can be reproduced here.

Table 19. Sample items from the Folstein Mini-Mental State Examination
Orientation to time
"What is the date?"
Registration
"Listen carefully. I am going to say three words. You say them back after I stop. Ready? Here they are . . .
APPLE (pause), PENNY (pause), TABLE (pause). Now repeat those words back to me." [Repeat up to five times, but score only the first trial.]
Naming
"What is this?" [Point to a pencil or pen.]
Reading
"Please read this and do what it says." [Show examinee the words on the stimulus form.]
CLOSE YOUR EYES

Depression history

 For this station, it is especially important to put the patient at ease and to be sensitive, tactful, and empathetic.

Before starting

- Introduce yourself to the patient.
- Explain that you are going to ask him some questions about his feelings, and ask for his consent to do this.
- Ensure that he is comfortable.
- Unless this information has been provided, ask for his name, age, and occupation.

The interview

- First ask open questions about the patient's current mood, listening attentively and gently encouraging him to open up.
- Ask about the onset of illness, and about its triggers and causes.

Ensure that you ask about:

- The core features of depression:
  - depressed mood
  - loss of interest
  - fatiguability
- Other common features of depression:
  - poor concentration
  - poor self-esteem and self-confidence
  - guilt
  - pessimism
- The somatic features of depression:
  - sleep disturbance
  - early morning waking
  - morning depression
  - loss of appetite and/or weight loss
  - loss of libido
  - anhedonia
  - agitation and/or retardation
- Screen for possible anxiety, obsessions, hallucinations, delusions, and mania.
- Take brief past medical, drug, and family history. Remember that drugs and alcohol are a common cause of depression.
- Assess the severity of the illness and its effect on the patient's life.

 Ask about suicidal ideation (also see Station 42: Suicide risk assessment). You may fail this station if you don't!

After finishing

- Ask the patient if there is anything he might add that you have forgotten to ask about.
- Thank him and offer a further course of action.

Suicide risk assessment

And so it was I entered the broken world
To trace the visionary company of love, its voice
An instant in the wind (I know not whither hurled)
But not for long to hold each desperate choice.

From *Broken Tower*, by Hart Crane (b. 1899; d. 1932, by suicide)

Before starting

- Introduce yourself to the patient.
- Establish rapport.

The assessment

Ask about:

- The history of the current episode of self-harm (if any):
  - what was the precipitant for the attempt?
  - was it planned?
  - what was the method of self-harm, and did he expect this to be lethal?
  - did he make a will or leave a suicide note?
  - was he alone?
  - was he intoxicated?
  - did he take any precautions against discovery?
  - did he seek help after the attempt?
  - how did he feel when help arrived?
- Assess risk factors for suicide:
  - previous suicide attempt(s)
  - recent life crisis
  - male sex, especially if between the ages of 25–44
  - divorced, widowed, or single
  - unemployed or in certain occupations, e.g. medicine, farming
  - poor level of social support
  - physical illness
  - psychiatric illness
  - substance misuse
  - family history of depression, substance misuse, or suicide
- Mental state: assess current mood and exclude psychosis.
- Will he be returning to the same situation? What has changed?
- Ask about current suicidal ideation. Has he made any plans?

After the assessment

- Thank the patient.
- Summarise your findings, state the patient's suicide risk, and suggest a plan of action (e.g. further investigations, psychiatric assessment, crisis team, hospitalisation …).

Alcohol history

Before starting

- Introduce yourself to the patient.
- Establish rapport.
- Explain to the patient that you would like to ask him some questions to evaluate his drinking habits, and ask for his consent to this. As he may be reluctant to give his consent, it is important that you be particularly gentle and tactful.

The alcohol history

Ask about:

- Alcohol intake:
  - amount
  - type
  - place
  - time
- Features of alcohol dependence:
  1. compulsion to drink
  2. primacy of drinking over other activities
  3. stereotyped pattern of drinking, e.g. narrowing of drinking repertoire
  4. increased tolerance to alcohol
  5. withdrawal symptoms, e.g. anxiety, sweating, tremor ('the shakes'), nausea, fits, *delirium tremens*
  6. relief drinking to avoid withdrawal symptoms
  7. reinstatement after abstinence

Medical history

Ask about depression and the common medical complications of alcohol abuse, e.g. peptic ulceration, pancreatitis, ischaemic heart disease, liver disease, peripheral neuropathy.

Drug history

Note that:

- Illicit drug use is common in alcoholics.
- Alcohol potentiates the effects of certain drugs such as phenytoin.

Family history

Social history

Cover employment, housing, marital problems, financial problems, and legal (forensic) problems.

After finishing

- Give the patient feedback on his drinking habits (e.g. number of units drunk versus recommended number of units) and, if appropriate, suggest ways for him to cut down his alcohol use.
- Ask him if he has any questions or concerns.
- Thank him for his cooperation.

One unit	One unit	One unit	One unit	One unit
1/2 pint of ordinary strength beer, lager or cider	1 very small glass of wine	1 single measure of spirits	1 small glass of sherry	1 single measure of aperitifs

Figure 33. Equivalences for one unit of alcohol. Note that one bottle of wine is equivalent to approximately 10 units, and one bottle of spirits to approximately 30 units.

Eating disorders history

Before starting

- Introduce yourself to the patient.
- Explain that you are going to ask some questions about her eating habits, and ask for her consent to do this.
- Ensure that she is comfortable.
- If this information is not provided, ask for her name, age, and occupation.

The history

Weight and perception of weight

Determine:

- Her current weight and height.
- The amount of weight that she has lost, and over what period.
- Whether the weight loss has been intentional.
- Whether she still considers that she is overweight.
- How often she weighs herself/looks at herself in the mirror.

Diet and compensatory behaviours

Ask about:

- Amount and type of food eaten in an average day.
- Binge eating.
- Vomiting.
- The use of laxatives, purgatives, diuretics, appetite suppressants, and stimulants.
- Physical exercise.

Other

Ask about:

- Menstrual periods.
- Effect on patient's life:
  - relationships
  - medical complications, e.g. anaemia, peptic ulceration, constipation
  - psychiatric complications, especially substance misuse, depression, and self harm
- Past medical, drug, and family history (briefly and only if you have time left).

After finishing

- Ask the patient if there is anything she might add that you have forgotten to ask about.
- Determine the patient's level of insight into her problem.
- Thank the patient, offer feedback, and suggest a further course of action, e.g. informant history from the mother, physical examination, investigations, dietary advice, psychotherapy, antidepressants, hospitalisation.

Table 20.   Anorexia nervosa vs. bulimia nervosa

DSM-IV diagnostic criteria

Anorexia

A.   Refusal to maintain normal body weight at more than 85% of expected body weight.

B.   Intense fear of gaining weight or becoming fat.

C.   Disturbed perception of body weight or shape.

D.   In postmenarchal females, amenorrhoea for at least three consecutive cycles (if not on the oral contraceptive pill).

Bulimia

A.   Recurrent episodes of binge eating.

B.   Recurrent inappropriate compensatory behaviour to prevent weight gain.

C.   Episodes of binge eating and compensatory behaviour occur at least twice a week for a period of 3 months.

D.   Self-evaluation is unduly influenced by body shape and weight.

E.   Disturbance does not occur exclusively during periods of anorexia nervosa.

Capacity and its assessment

In this station, you may be asked to carry out a formalised assessment of competence to decide on the ability of a patient to give informed consent (see *Station 111*). Alternatively, you may simply be asked to discuss the subject.

The first thing to note is that the terms capacity and competence are often used interchangeably but, strictly speaking, capacity is the legal presumption that adult persons have the ability to make decisions, whereas competence is a clinical determination of a patient's ability to make decisions about his treatment.

Issues about capacity frequently arise in three groups of patients: children and adolescents, patients with learning difficulties, and patients with mental illness. A person has capacity so long as he has the ability to understand and retain relevant information for long enough to reach a *reasoned* decision, **regardless of the actual decision reached**. An adult person should be presumed to have the competence to make a particular decision until a judgement about capacity can be made. This judgement can only be made about present capacity, not about past or future capacity, and it should only be made for a specific decision, as different decisions require different levels of capacity. If capacity is lacking or cannot be established (e.g. in an emergency situation), the doctor in charge has the responsibility to act in the best interests of the patient, although it is good practice for him to involve colleagues, carers, and relatives in the decision-making. In difficult situations or if there are differences of opinion about the patient's best interests, the doctor should consult a senior colleague or seek legal advice. In England and Wales, the Mental Capacity Act 2005 provides for a Court of Protection to help with difficult decisions.

Assessing capacity

1. Ensure that the patient understands:
    *   what the intervention is
    *   why the intervention is being proposed
    *   the alternatives to the intervention, including no intervention
    *   the principal benefits and risks of the intervention and of its alternatives
    *   the consequences of the intervention and of its alternatives
2. Ensure that the patient retains the information for long enough to weigh it in the balance and reach a reasoned decision, whatever that decision might be. In some cases, the patient may not have the cognitive ability or emotional maturity to reach a reasoned decision, or may be unduly affected by mental illness.
3. Ensure that the patient is not subject to coercion or threat.

It is important to bear in mind that a patient's capacity can be enhanced by, for example:

*   making your explanations easier to understand, e.g. using diagrams
*   seeing the patient at his best time of day
*   seeing the patient with a friend or relative
*   improving the patient's environment, e.g. finding a quiet side-room
*   adjusting the patient's medication, e.g. decreasing the dose of sedative drugs

In England and Wales, the Mental Capacity Act 2005 provides for an Independent Mental Capacity Advocate (IMCA) service to help people who have no 'intimate support network'.

Hearing and the ear examination

Before starting

- Introduce yourself to the patient.
- Explain the examination and ask for his consent to carry it out.
- Sit him so that he is facing you and ensure that he is comfortable.

The history

- Name, age, and occupation, if this information has not already been provided.
- Ask the patient if there has been any loss of hearing.

If there has been loss of hearing, assess its:

- Characteristics (bilaterality, onset, duration, severity, impact on the patient's life).
- Associated features (tinnitus, vertigo, pain, discharge, weight loss).
- Possible causes (trauma, infection, antibiotics, family history).
- Impact on the patient's life.

The examination

Hearing

Test hearing by whispering into the ear at various distances, whilst distracting or occluding the other ear. As whispering into people's ears may no longer be considered politically correct, you may prefer rubbing your fingers together instead.

Tuning fork tests

 Use a 512 Hz tuning fork, and not the larger 128 Hz or 256 Hz tuning forks used for neurological examinations.

- The Rinne test. Place the base of the vibrating tuning fork on the mastoid process of each ear. Once the patient can no longer 'hear' the vibration, move the tuning fork in front of the ear. If the tuning fork can be heard, air conduction is better than bone conduction, and there is therefore no conductive hearing loss. The test is said to be *positive*. If the tuning fork cannot be heard, there is a conductive hearing loss, and the test is said to be *negative*.

 The false negative Rinne test: if the Rinne test is performed on a deaf ear, it may appear negative because the vibration is transmitted to the opposite ear.

- The Weber test. Place the vibrating tuning fork in the midline of the skull. If hearing is normal, or if hearing loss is symmetrical, the vibration should be heard equally in both ears.

Note:

- If there is conductive deafness in one ear, the vibration is best heard *in that same ear* (since there is no background interference).
- If there is sensorineural deafness in one ear, the vibration is best heard in the other ear.

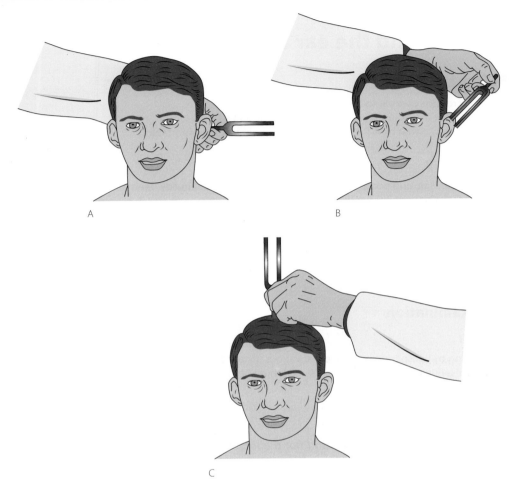

Figure 34. The Rinne (A, B) and Weber (C) tests.

Auroscopy

- Examine the pinnae for size, shape, deformities, pre-auricular sinuses.
- Look behind the ears for any scars.
- Palpate the pre-auricular, post-auricular, and infra-auricular lymph nodes.
- Affix a speculum of appropriate size onto the auroscope.
- Gently pull the ear so as to straighten the ear canal and, holding the auroscope like a pen, introduce it into the external auditory meatus.

 If examining the right ear, use your right hand to hold the auroscope. If examining the left ear, use your left hand.

- Through the auroscope, inspect the ear canal (otitis externa, exotoses, wax) and the tympanic membrane (normal anatomy, effusions, cholesteatomata, perforations, grommets).

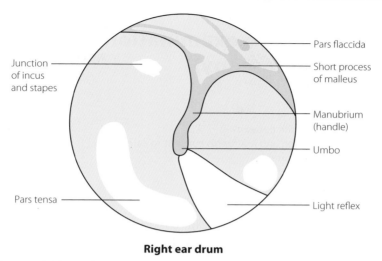

Right ear drum

Figure 35. The normal right ear drum.

After examining the ear

- Ask the patient if he has any questions or concerns.
- Thank the patient.
- Summarise your findings and offer a differential diagnosis, e.g. ear wax, otitis media, perforated ear drum.

Figure 36. Otitis media with effusion.

Reproduced with permission from Michael Saunders, Bristol Royal Infirmary.

Station 47

Vision and the eye examination (including fundoscopy)

Before starting

- Introduce yourself to the patient.
- Explain the examination and ask for his consent to carry it out.
- Ensure that he is comfortable.

The examination

1. Visual acuity

- *Snellen chart.* Assess each eye individually, correcting for any refractive errors (glasses, pinhole). If the patient cannot read the Snellen chart, either move him closer or ask him to count fingers. If he fails to count fingers, test whether he can see hand movements and, if he cannot, test whether he can see light.
- *Test types* (or fine print). Assess each eye individually, correcting for any refractive errors.
- *Ishihara plates.* Indicate that you could use Ishihara plates to test colour vision specifically.

2. Visual fields

- *Confrontation test.* Sit at 1 m from the patient. Cover your left eye with your left hand and ask the patient to cover his right eye and to fix his gaze upon your right eye. Starting at a distance, bring an equidistant moving finger into each of his upper and lower temporal fields. Then change hands and test his upper and lower nasal fields. Compare the patient's visual field to your own. Test the other eye.
- *Visual inattention test.* Ask the patient to fix his gaze upon you and simultaneously bring a moving finger into each of the patient's right and left visual fields. In some parietal lobe lesions, only an ipsilateral finger is perceived by the patient.
- *Mapping of central visual field defects.* Indicate that you could use a red pin to delineate the patient's blind spot and any central visual field defects.

3. Pupillary reflexes

- *Inspection.* Inspect the pupils for size and shape.
- *Pupillary reflexes.* Ask the patient to fixate on a distant object and, using a pen torch, test the direct and consensual pupillary reflexes. If the consensual pupillary reflex is absent, there is a relative afferent pupillary defect, or Marcus Gunn pupil.
- *Accommodation reflex.* Test the accommodation reflex by asking the patient to focus on a distant object and then on a finger held at 30 cm from his face.

4. Eye movements

- *Inspection.* Look for a squint.
- *Cover test.* Indicate that you could perform a cover test to look for a concomitant squint.
- *Eye movements.* Fix the patient's head and ask him to track your finger through an 'H' pattern. Ask him to report any double vision.
- *Nystagmus.* Look out for nystagmus at the extremes of gaze. You can do this as part of eye movements or separately by fixing the patient's head and asking him to track your finger through a cross pattern.

5. Fundoscopy

Explain the procedure, mentioning that it may be uncomfortable. Darken the room and ask the patient to fixate on a distant object (or to 'look over my shoulder'). State to the examiner that, ideally, the pupils should have been dilated using a solution of 1% cyclopentolate.

- *Red reflex.* Test from a distance of 1 m by looking through the ophthalmoscope. An absent red reflex is usually caused by a cataract.
- *Fundoscopy.* Use your right eye to examine the patient's right eye, and your left eye to examine the patient's left eye. If you use your left eye to examine the patient's right eye, you may appear more caring than the examiner might like to see. Look at the optic nerve head, the vessels, and the macula. Describe any features according to protocol, e.g. *There are soft exudates at 3 o'clock, two disc diameters away from the disc.*

 If the station is examining fundoscopy alone, the patient is likely to be replaced by a model in which the retinas are very easy to visualise. Before the exam, it is a good idea to look at as many retinas as you can, both in patients and in textbooks/on the internet. Conditions likely to be examined include cataract, age-related macular degeneration, hypertensive retinopathy, diabetic retinopathy, glaucoma, central retinal artery and central retinal vein occlusion, and papilloedema.

After the examination

- Ask the patient if he has any questions or concerns.
- Thank the patient.
- Summarise your findings and offer a differential diagnosis.

Table 21. Common findings on fundoscopy	
Cataract	Absent red reflex, on approaching the ophthalmoscope the lens may look like cracked ice
Age-related macular degeneration	Drusen (characteristic yellow deposits) in the macula, exudative changes resulting from blood and fluid under the macula
Hypertensive retinopathy	Stage I: arteriolar narrowing and tortuosity
	Stage II: AV nicking, silver-wiring
	Stage III: dot, blot, and flame haemorrhages, microaneurysms, soft exudates (cotton-wool spots), hard exudates
	Stage IV: papilloedema
Diabetic retinopathy	Background: microaneurysms, macular oedema, hard exudates, haemorrhages
	Pre-proliferative: cotton-wool spots, venous beading
	Proliferative: neovascularisation, vitreous haemorrhage
Glaucoma	Increased cup to disc ratio, haemorrhages
Central retinal artery occlusion	Pale retina with swelling or oedema, markedly decreased vascularity, cherry red spot in the central fovea
Central retinal vein occlusion	Widespread haemorrhages throughout the retina with swelling and oedema, sometimes described as a 'stormy sunset' – something to look out for on your elective
Papilloedema	Blurring of disc margins, cupping and swelling of the disc, haemorrhages, exudates, distended veins

Figure 37. Findings on fundoscopy of the right eye.
1.   Normal.
2.   Senile macular degeneration.
3.   Hypertensive retinopathy.
4.   Pre-proliferative diabetic retinopathy.
5.   Central retinal vein occlusion.
6.   Papilloedema.

Smell and the nose examination

Specifications: This station may involve a model of a nose in lieu of a patient.

Before starting

- Introduce yourself to the patient.
- Explain the examination and ask him for his consent to carry it out.
- Position him so that he is facing you.
- Ensure that he is comfortable.

The history

- Briefly establish the nature of the problem.
- If there is obstruction of the nasal passages, determine its:
  - characteristics (nasal passage affected, onset, duration, timing, severity)
  - associated symptoms (facial pain, inflammation, itching, rhinorrhoea, sneezing, snoring, anosmia)
  - possible causes (asthma, hay fever, other allergies, trauma, surgery, other)
  - impact on everyday life

The examination

Inspection

- Observe the external appearance of the nose from the front, from the side, and from above. Look for evidence of deformity, inflammation, nasal discharge, skin disease, and scars.
- Examine the nasal vestibule, anterior end of the septum, and anterior ends of the inferior turbinates. Do this first by elevating the tip of the nose, and then with the help of a Thudicum speculum and torch.
- Look into the mouth.

Otoscopy

- Use an otoscope in conjunction with a Thudicum speculum to assess the nasal septum and the inferior and middle turbinates. Look for septal deviation, mucosal inflammation, polyps, and foreign objects.

 A more detailed view of the nasal cavities can be obtained using a flexible (fibre-optic) nasendoscope.

Nasal airflow

- Ask the patient to breathe out through his nose onto a mirror or cold tongue depressor positioned under the nose. If the nasal passages are not obstructed, there should be condensation under both nostrils.
- Assess inspiratory flow by occluding one nostril and asking the patient to sniff. Repeat for the other side.

Smell

- Assess sense of smell by asking the patient to identify fragrances from a series of bottles containing different odours.

After examining the nose

- Ask the patient if he has any questions or concerns.
- Thank the patient.
- Summarise your findings and offer a differential diagnosis.

Figure 38. Nasal polyp.

Reproduced from www.askdrshah.com with permission from Dr Rajesh Shah.

Lump in the neck examination

Before starting

- Introduce yourself to the patient.
- Explain the examination and ask for his consent to carry it out.
- Ask him to expose his neck and upper body.
- Sit him in a chair.

The examination

Inspection

- Inspect the patient generally, in particular looking for any signs of thyroid disease. The age and sex of the patient has an important bearing on the differential diagnosis of a goitre.
- Inspect the neck, looking for asymmetry, scars, or other lesions.

 A goitre, or enlarged thyroid gland, is seen as a swelling below the cricoid cartilage, on either side of the trachea.

- Ask the patient to take a sip of water. The following structures move upon swallowing: thyroid gland, thyroid cartilage, cricoid cartilage, thyroglossal cyst, lymph nodes.
- Ask him to stick his tongue out. A midline swelling which moves upwards when the tongue is protruded is a thyroglossal cyst.
- Position yourself behind him and inspect for exophthalmos from above.

Palpation

- Ask him if there is any tenderness in the neck area.
- Putting one hand on either side of his neck, examine the anterior and posterior triangles of the neck with your fingertips. For any mass, try to determine its size, consistency, and fixity.
- Palpate the thyroid gland. Try to determine its size, symmetry, and consistency, and whether it is tender to touch. Note that the normal thyroid gland is often not palpable.
- Palpate the cervical lymph nodes.
- Palpate for tracheal deviation in the suprasternal notch (see *Station 16: Respiratory system examination*), which features in *The English Patient* as an erogenous zone.

Percussion

- Percuss for the dullness of a retrosternal goitre over the sternum and upper chest.

Auscultation

- Auscultate over the thyroid for bruits. Ask the patient to hold his breath as you listen; a soft bruit is sometimes heard in thyrotoxicosis.

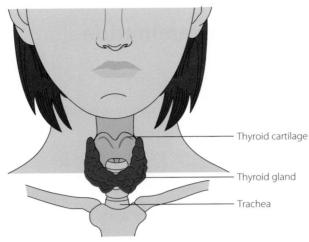

Thyroid cartilage

Thyroid gland

Trachea

Figure 39. Anatomy of the normal thyroid gland.

After the examination

- Help the patient to put his clothes back on.
- Ensure that he is comfortable.
- Ask him if he has any questions or concerns.
- Thank him.
- Offer a diagnosis or differential diagnosis.
- Give suggestions for further management, e.g. thyroid function tests, thyroid antibodies, ultrasound examination of the thyroid, iodine thyroid scan, fine needle aspiration cytology.

Goitres and thyroid disease

Signs of **hyperthyroidism**: enlarged thyroid gland or thyroid nodules, thyroid bruit, hyperthermia, diaphoresis, dehydration, tremor, tachycardia, arrhythmia, congestive cardiac failure, onycholysis.

- Grave's disease (commonest cause of hyperthyroidism): uniformly enlarged smooth thyroid gland usually in a younger patient; lid retraction, lid lag, chemosis, periorbital oedema, proptosis, diplopia, pre-tibial myxoedema (non-pitting oedema and skin thickening, seen in <5% of cases), thyroid acropachy (finger clubbing, seen in <1% of cases).
- Toxic multinodular goitre: enlarged multinodular goitre in a middle-aged patient.
- Toxic nodule and de Quervain's thyroiditis are less common.

Signs of **hypothyrodism**: hypothermia and cold intolerance, weight gain, slowed speech and movements, hoarse voice, dry skin, hair loss, coarse facial features and facial puffiness, hypotension, bradycardia, and hyporeflexia.

- Hashimoto's thyroiditis (commonest cause of hypothyroidism): moderately enlarged rubbery thyroid gland, usually in a female patient aged 30–50 years; initial hyperthyroidism that progresses to hypothyroidism and, if untreated, to myxoedema.

[Note] Iodine deficiency can also cause a goitre but this is rarely seen in developed countries.

Figure 40. Eye signs in Grave's disease.
Reproduced from www.eyeplastics.net.

Most common conditions likely to come up in a neck examination station
Thyroglossal cyst
Toxic goitre: diffuse (Grave's disease), multinodular, toxic nodule (Plummer's disease)
Hashimoto's thyroiditis
Thyroid neoplasm
Enlarged lymph nodes
Physiological goitre of puberty or of pregnancy (or of both, these days)

Dermatological history

Before starting

- Introduce yourself to the patient.
- Explain that you are going to ask him some questions to uncover the nature of his skin problem, and ask for his consent to do this.
- Ensure that he is comfortable; if not, make sure that he is.

The history

- Name and age.

Presenting complaint

- Use an open question to ask the patient to describe his skin problem.

History of presenting complaint

Ask about:

- When, where, and how the problem started.
- What the initial lesions looked like and how they have evolved.
- Symptoms: especially, pain, pruritus, and bleeding.
- Aggravating factors such as sunlight, heat, soaps, etc.
- Relieving factors, including any treatments so far.
- Effect on everyday life.
- Details of previous episodes, if any.

Past medical history

- Previous skin disease.
- Atopy (asthma, allergic rhinitis, childhood eczema).
- Present and past medical illnesses.
- Surgery.

Drug history

- Prescribed and OTC/complementary medications, including topical applications such as gels and creams (including in the recent past).
- Cosmetics and moisturising creams (including in the recent past).
- Relationship of symptoms to use of medication.
- Allergies.

Family history

- Has anyone in the family had a similar problem?
- Medical history of parents, siblings, and children, focusing on skin problems.
- Sexual contacts.

Social history

- Occupation (in some detail, e.g. potential exposure to chemicals, similar symptoms in one or more colleagues). Does the skin problem improve during holiday periods?
- Hobbies (in some detail).
- Home circumstances.
- Alcohol use.
- Recent travel, especially to the tropics.

Systems review

(If appropriate.)

After taking the history

- Ask the patient if there is anything that he might add that you have forgotten to ask about.
- Thank the patient.
- Summarise your findings and offer a differential diagnosis.
- State that you should next like to carry out a dermatological examination.

Station 51

Dermatological examination

Before starting

- Introduce yourself to the patient.
- Explain the examination and ask for his consent to carry it out.
- Ask him to undress to his undergarments.
- Ensure that he is comfortable.
- Ask him to report any pain or discomfort during the examination.
- Ensure that there is adequate lighting.

The examination

- Describe the distribution of the lesions: are they generalised or localised, symmetrical or asymmetrical, affecting only certain areas, e.g. flexor or extensor surfaces. Make a point of looking at all parts of the body.
- Describe the morphology of the individual lesions, commenting upon their colour, size, shape, borders, elevation, and spatial relationship. Use precise dermatological terms. A glossary of dermatological terms can be found on the Molson Medical Informatics Student Projects website at http://sprojects.mmi.mcgill.ca/dermatology/terminology.htm.
- Note any secondary skin lesions such as scaling, lichenification, crusting, excoriation, erosion, ulceration, and scarring.
- Palpate the lesions (ask the patient if this is OK first). Assess their consistency. Do they blanch?
- Examine the finger nails and toe nails.
- Examine the hair and scalp.
- Examine the mucous membranes.
- Check for lymphadenopathy, if appropriate.
- Check the pedal pulses, if appropriate.

After the examination

- If appropriate, offer to help the patient to put his clothes back on.
- Thank the patient.
- Ensure that he is comfortable.
- Wash your hands.
- Summarise your findings and offer a differential diagnosis.

Most common conditions likely to come up in a skin examination station
Psoriasis
Eczema
Contact dermatitis
Acne vulgaris
Erythema nodosum
Malignant melanoma
Basal cell carcinoma
Squamous cell carcinoma

Figure 41. Basal cell carcinoma (BCC).

Reproduced from http://picasaweb.google.com/schalock.

Examiner's questions

Differentiating skin cancers

BCC (75% of skin cancers) most often looks like a pearly bump or nodule on sun-exposed areas of skin. Bleeding or crusting may develop in the centre of the tumour, as in the photograph above. In contrast, squamous cell carcinoma (SCC, 20% of all skin cancers) most often looks a red, scaling, thickened patch, sometimes with bleeding, crusting, or ulceration. Although less common than either BCC or SCC, malignant melanoma is more commonly fatal. Pigmented lesions of the skin should be suspected to be malignant melanomas if they are **a**symmetrical, if they have irregular **b**orders, if their **c**olour varies from one area to another, or if their **d**iameter is larger than that of a pencil eraser (6 mm). This is easily remembered as A, B, C, D.

Station 52

Advice on sun protection

 Read in conjunction with Station 110: Explaining skills.

Before starting

- Introduce yourself to the patient.
- Tell him what you are going to explain, and determine how much he already knows.

The advice

Explain that there are three types of ultraviolet radiation from the sun: UVA, UVB, and UVC.

- UVA and UVB can cause skin cancer.
- UVC does not reach the surface of the earth and is therefore of no concern.

Explain that, other than causing skin cancer, UV radiation can also cause the skin to burn and (horror!) to age prematurely.

UV levels depend on a number of factors such as the time of day, time of year, latitude, altitude, cloud cover, and ozone cover.

Explain that there are four principal methods of protecting against the sun's rays:

1. Avoid the outdoors. The sun's rays are most direct around midday and so one should avoid being outdoors from around 11 am to 3 pm.
2. Seek shade.
3. Cover up (clothing should include a wide-brimmed hat and sunglasses that conform to British Standard 2724).
4. Use sunscreen.
   - A sunscreen's star rating is a measure of its level of protection against UVA.
   - A sunscreen's sun protection factor is a measure of its level of protection against UVB.
   - Use a sunscreen that has a star rating of at least three stars *** and an SPF of at least 15.
   - The sunscreen should be applied thickly over all sun-exposed areas, and re-applied regularly.

 It is important that you explain that sunscreens should not simply be used as a means of spending more time in the sun.

Finally advise the patient to report any moles that change in size, shape, colour, or texture.

After giving the advice

- Summarise the information and ensure that the patient has understood it.
- Tell them that, if anything, they can remember 'Slip, slap, slop' – slip on some clothes, slap on a hat, and slop on sunscreen.
- Ask the patient if he has any questions or concerns.
- Give the patient a leaflet on sun protection.

Paediatric history

General points:

- As a rule of thumb, the older the child the more he should be involved in the history-taking process.
- Observe the child's behaviour as you take the history.
- The parent's concerns and the child's concerns are likely to differ: try as much as possible to address both.

Before starting

- Introduce yourself to the parent and child (in that order).
- Explain that you are going to ask some questions and obtain consent to do this.
- Ensure that the patient is comfortable; younger children may need some toys to keep them distracted.

The history

- Ask the age, sex, and preferred name of the child.
- Confirm the relationship of the accompanying adult.

Presenting complaint and history of presenting complaint

- Ask about the nature of the presenting complaint and how it has affected the child's daily routine. Start by using open questions and then explore the symptoms as you might in any other history. Ask about onset, duration, previous episodes, pain, associated symptoms (e.g. nausea, vomiting, diarrhoea, urinary frequency, constipation, altered consciousness), and treatments.

 Do not under any circumstances denigrate, or omit to address, the parent's concerns.

Systems review

- The major systems should be covered briefly, placing the emphasis on areas of particular relevance.
    - *General health*: liveliness, change in behaviour, ability to recover from a minor illness.
    - *ENT*: sore throat, earache, infections, deafness, nose bleeds.
    - *CVS and RS*: breathing problems (feeding problems in young infants), shortness of breath, exercise tolerance, colour changes (blue attacks, pallor), wheeze, croup, stridor, cough, chest infections, tiredness, heart murmurs.
    - *GIS*: weight gain, feeding, vomiting, diarrhoea, constipation, jaundice, abdominal pain.
    - *GUS*: frequency, discharge, enuresis.
    - *NS*: headaches, fits, visual disturbances, balance and coordination, muscle problems.
    - *MSS*: limps, joint stiffness, pain, swelling, redness.
    - *Skin*: rash, eczema.

Past medical history

Similar problems in the past?

Ask about these topics if you think that they might be relevant to the child's presenting complaint.

- Medical problems (epilepsy, diabetes, asthma, etc.)
- Surgery.
- Birth history:
  - maternal obstetric history (illnesses or infections during pregnancy, blood pressure, foetal growth, drugs during pregnancy, e.g. anti-convulsants, narcotics, smoking, alcohol)
  - mode of delivery and any problems
  - gestation at delivery
  - birth weight
  - problems after birth and admission to Special Care Baby Unit
- Developmental milestones (smiling, sitting, walking and talking – see *Station 54: Developmental assessment*).
- Feeding (breast, bottle, how long, how much).
- Sleeping patterns.
- Childhood illnesses.
- Immunisations.

Drug history

- Prescribed and over-the-counter medications.
- Allergies.

Family history

- Health of parents and siblings.
- Congenital/genetic abnormalities. (*"Are there any illnesses that run in the family?"*)
- Cosanguinity.

Social history

- Parental occupation.
- Details of home life, siblings.
- Behaviour at home and at school.
- Pets and smokers in the home (if relevant).

After taking the history

- Ask the parent if there is anything that he/she might add that you have forgotten to ask about.
- Ask the parent and child if they have any specific questions or concerns.
- Thank the parent and child.
- Summarise your findings and offer a differential diagnosis.

Most common conditions likely to come up in a paediatric history station
Respiratory conditions, e.g. asthma, upper respiratory tract infection
Headache
Behavioural problems, e.g. enuresis
Fits, e.g. febrile convulsions, epilepsy
Childhood infections/rashes and immunisation compliance (see *Station 62: Child immunisation programme*).

Developmental assessment

Development in the early years of life is fairly consistent from child to child and any significant deviation from this pattern is thus a reliable marker of pathology.

The four parameters by which development is assessed

1. Gross motor skills
2. Vision and fine movement
3. Hearing and language
4. Social behaviour

Key ages for developmental assessment

1. Newborn
2. Supine infant (1.5–2 months)
3. Sitting infant (6–9 months)
4. Toddler (18–24 months)
5. Communicating child (3–4 years)

The developmental assessment

Specifications: This station may require you to carry out a developmental assessment or watch a short video and answer some questions about it.

The developmental assessment is usually performed alongside a general history, so many of the subject headings are the same as in *Station 53: Paediatric history*. Remember to tailor the assessment to the age of the child and that much of the assessment can and should be carried out by observation alone.

Before starting

- Introduce yourself to the parent and child.
- Explain that you are going to ask some questions and obtain consent to do this.
- Ensure that the child is comfortable; younger children may need toys to keep them distracted.
- Ask for the child's red book.

The assessment

- Ask for the age, sex, and preferred name of the child.

Presenting complaint and history of presenting complaint

- Ask about the nature of the presenting complaint and its effects on the child's daily routine. Use open questions.

Table 22. Average age for the acquisition of key milestones

	Motor skills	Vision and fine movement	Hearing and language	Social behaviour
Newborn	Symmetrical movements, limbs flexed, head lag on pulling up	Looks at light/faces in direct line of vision	Startles to noises/voices	Responds to parents
Supine infant (1.5–2 months)	Raises head in prone position	Tracks objects	Cries, coos, grunts	Smiles at faces
Sitting infant (6–9 months)	6/12: sits unsupported 8/12: crawls 9/12: stands supported	6/12: 'palmar grasp' 6–7/12: transfers objects	Babbles	Develops stranger and separation anxiety. Likes playing 'peek-a-boo'
Toddler (18–24 months)	12/12: stands unsupported and makes first steps 15/12: walks 24/12: climbs stairs	12/12: 'pincer grip' 16/12: uses spoon or fork	12/12: vocabulary of 1–3 words 24/12: vocabulary of >200 words; makes phrases	Is prone to temper tantrums
Communicating child (3–4 years)	Stands on one leg. Jumps. Pedals tricycle	Mature pencil grip. Draws a circle and a cross	Makes complete sentences	Plays co-operatively with other children. Imitates parents. Achieves urinary continence

Developmental/past medical history

- Birth history:
  - maternal obstetric history
  - mode of delivery and any problems
  - gestation at delivery
  - birth weight
  - problems after birth and admission to Special Care Baby Unit
  - initial feedings
  - medical problems, childhood illnesses, immunisations
- Key milestones:
  - smiling
  - sitting
  - walking
  - talking
- Current abilities:
  - motor skills
  - vision and fine movement
  - language and hearing
  - social behaviour

Systems review
Drug history
Family history
Social history

After the assessment

- Ask the parent if there is anything he/she might add that you have forgotten to ask about.
- Ask the parent if he/she has any specific questions or concerns.
- Thank the parent and child.
- Summarise your findings and offer a differential diagnosis.

Most common conditions likely to come up in a developmental assessment station
Late walker
Developmental disorder, e.g. autism
Mental retardation
Emotional disorder, e.g. enuresis, elective mutism, sleep disorders
Behavioural disorder, e.g. conduct disorder, ADHD

Neonatal examination

Specifications: A mannequin in lieu of a baby. The baby's 'mother' is also in the room.

Before starting

- Introduce yourself to the mother, explain the examination, and ask her for her consent to carry it out.
- Wash your hands.
- Ask the mother about:
  - complications of the pregnancy, if any
  - type of delivery
  - the baby's gestational age at the time of birth
  - the baby's birth weight
  - the baby's feeding, urination, and defaecation
  - any concerns that she might have

The examination

Figure 42. Neonatal examination, general order of the examination.

General inspection

Note colour, position, tone, movements, skin abnormalities, and any other obvious abnormalities. Are there any signs of respiratory distress?

Head

- Palpate the anterior and posterior fontanelles.
- Measure the head circumference.

Face

- Inspect the face for dysmorphological features.
- Check the patency of the ears and nostrils.

- Using an ophthalmoscope, test the red reflex and pupillary reflexes.
- Test eye movements (squint).
- Elicit the rooting reflex by lightly touching a corner of the baby's mouth.
- Introduce a finger into the baby's mouth and feel the palate (cleft palate).
- Examine the palate using a torch and spatula.

Chest

- Take the radial and femoral pulses, one after the other and then both at the same time (radiofemoral delay).
- Listen to the heart using the bell of your stethoscope.
- Listen to the lungs using the diaphragm of your stethoscope. Turn the infant over and listen over the back. The respiratory rate should be less than 60 breaths per minute.

Back

- Examine the spine, focusing on the sacral pit (neural tube defects).
- Check the position and patency of the anus.

Abdomen

- Inspect the abdomen and the umbilical cord.
- Palpate the abdomen.
- Palpate specifically for the spleen, liver, and kidneys (thumb in front, finger in the loin).
- Feel for the femoral pulses.
- Examine the genitalia, in male infants note the position of the urethral meatus (hypospadias), ask about the urine stream, and feel for the testicles (undescended testes).

Hips

- Abduct the hips (Ortolani test, detects relocation of a dislocated hip).
- Next, adduct them whilst applying pressure with your thumbs (Barlow test, detects a dislocated hip).

Ortolani test

Barlow test

Figure 43. The Ortolani and Barlow tests.

Arms and hands

- Inspect the arms and hands, paying particular attention to the palmar creases (trisomy).
- Count the number of fingers on each hand.

Feet

- Inspect the feet and test their range of movement.
- Count the number of toes on each foot.

Posture and reflexes

- Test head lag by lying the baby supine and pulling up his upper body by the arms.
- Hold the baby prone – the head should lie above the midline.
- Test the Moro reflex by lifting the head and shoulders and then suddenly dropping them back – the arms and legs should abduct and extend symmetrically, and then adduct and flex (NB: some examiners may prefer that you did not test the Moro reflex).
- Test the grasp reflex by placing a finger in the baby's hand.

Figure 44. Eliciting the Moro reflex.

After the neonatal examination

- State that you would also measure and weigh the baby.
- Summarise your findings.
- Reassure the mother, and tell her that you are going to have the baby examined by a senior colleague.

The six-week surveillance review

Specifications: A mannequin in lieu of a baby.

Before starting

- Introduce yourself to the parent.
- Explain the nature of the examination and obtain consent.
- Ask for the parent-held record.

The history

- Ask for the exact age, sex, and preferred name of the child.

Main concerns

- Ask if the parent has any specific concerns.

Past medical history

- Birth history:
  - pregnancy
  - gestation
  - delivery
  - birth weight
  - neonatal history
- Present health:
  - current health status
  - medication
  - social history

The examination

PART 1 – DEVELOPMENTAL ASSESSMENT

Motor skills

- Symmetrical limb movements.
- Head lag.

Vision and fine movement

- Looks at light/faces.
- Follows an object.

Hearing and language

- Responds to noises/voices.
- Normal cry.
- Ask parent if he/she is concerned about the baby's hearing.

Social behaviour

- Smiles responsively.

PART 2 – PHYSICAL EXAMINATION

Growth

- Weight.
- Length.
- Head circumference.
- Plot findings on a centile chart.

Head

- Palpate the fontanelles.

Face

- Eyes: red reflex, papillary reflexes, and eye movements (squints).
- Ears.
- Mouth – use a pen torch.

Chest

- Feel for the radial and femoral pulses.
- Auscultate the heart.
- Auscultate the lungs.

Back

- Examine the spine, particularly the sacral pit.

Abdomen

- Inspect and palpate the abdomen.
- Examine the external genitalia.

Hips

- Abduct the hips (Ortolani test, see *Figure 43*).
- Next, adduct them whilst applying pressure with your thumbs (Barlow test, see *Figure 43*).

After the surveillance review

- Discuss your findings with the parent.
- Use the opportunity for health promotion, e.g. immunisations, accident prevention, services available for the parents of young children.
- Elicit any remaining concerns that the parent may have.
- Thank the parent.

Paediatric examination: cardiovascular system

If you are asked to examine the cardiovascular system of a younger child (an unlikely event), be prepared to change the order of your examination and to modify your technique as appropriate. For example, you may need to examine the child on his parent's knees or auscultate his heart as soon as he stops crying. As in all paediatric stations, the quality of your rapport with the child will be of considerable importance.

Before starting

- Introduce yourself to the child and the parent.
- Explain the examination and ask for consent to carry it out.
- Position the child at 45 degrees, and ask him to remove his top(s).
- Ensure that he is comfortable.

The examination

General inspection

- From the end of the couch, inspect the child carefully, looking for any obvious abnormalities in his general appearance.
- Does the child look his age? Ask to look at the growth chart.
- Is he breathless or cyanosed?
- Look around the child for clues such as a oxygen, PEFR meter, inhalers, etc.
- Inspect the precordium and the chest for any scars and pulsations. A median sternotomy or thoracotomy scar under the axillae may indicate the repair of a congenital heart defect such as a patent ductus arteriosus or a ventricular septal defect.

Inspection and examination of the hands

- Take both hands and assess them for:
  - colour and temperature
  - clubbing
  - nail signs
- Determine the rate, rhythm, and character of both radial pulses (in younger infants, the brachial pulses). Take both femoral pulses at the same time to exclude a radiofemoral delay (coarctation of the aorta).
- Indicate that you would record the blood pressure in both arms. If you are asked to record the blood pressure, remember to use a cuff of appropriate size.

Table 23. Normal pulse rates in children	
Age in years	Pulse (beats per minute)
< 1	100–160
2–4	90–140
4–10	80–140
> 10	65–100

Inspection and examination of the head and neck

- Inspect the conjunctiva for signs of anaemia.
- Inspect the mouth and tongue for signs of central cyanosis.
- Assess the jugular venous pressure (difficult in very young infants).
- Locate the carotid pulse and assess its character.

Palpation of the heart

 Ask the child if he has any pain in the chest.

- Determine the location and character of the apex beat. In children (up to 8 years), this is found in the fourth intercostal space in the mid-clavicular line.
- Palpate the precordium for thrills and heaves.

Auscultation of the heart

 Warm up the diaphragm of your stethoscope.

- Listen for heart sounds, additional sounds, and murmurs. Using the stethoscope's diaphragm, listen in:
    - the *aortic* area
    - the *pulmonary* area
    - the *tricuspid* area
    - the *mitral* area

(See *Station 12, Figure 9.*)

- Any murmur heard must be classified according to:
    - timing
    - grading
    - site
    - radiation

Innocent murmurs are common in childhood
Innocent murmurs are:
• Systolic.
• Low-grade.
• Heard over only a relatively small area.
• Asymptomatic.

Chest examination

Auscultate the bases of the lungs and check for sacral oedema.

Abdominal examination

Palpate the abdomen to exclude ascities and/or an enlarged liver. Note that the liver edge can usually be palpated in younger infants.

Peripheral pulses

Feel the temperature of the feet, palpate the femoral pulses, and check for pedal oedema.

After the examination

- Cover the child.
- Ask the child and parent if they have any questions or concerns.
- Thank the child and parent.
- Indicate that you would test the urine, examine the retina with an ophthalmoscope and, if appropriate, order some key investigations, e.g. a CXR, ECG, echocardiogram.
- Summarise your findings and offer a differential diagnosis.

Most common conditions likely to come up in a paediatric examination: cardiovascular system station
Ventricular septal defect (VSD)
Patent ductus arteriosus (PDA)
Atrial septal defect (ASD)
Pulmonary stenosis
Aortic stenosis/hypertrophic obstructive cardiomyopathy (HOCM)
Coarctation of the aorta

Paediatric examination: respiratory system

If you are asked to examine the respiratory system of a younger child (an unlikely event), be prepared to change the order of your examination and to modify your technique as appropriate. For example, you may need to examine the child on his parent's knees or auscultate his chest as soon as he stops crying. As in all paediatric stations, the quality of your rapport with the child will be of considerable importance.

Before starting

- Introduce yourself to the child and parent.
- Explain the examination and ask for consent to carry it out.
- Position the child at 45 degrees, and ask him to remove his top(s).
- Ensure that he is comfortable.

The examination

General inspection

- From the end of the couch inspect the child carefully, looking for any obvious abnormalities in his general appearance.
- Does the child look his age? Ask to look at the growth chart.
- Is he breathless or cyanosed?
- Is his breathing audible?
- Note the rate, depth, and regularity of his breathing.
- Look around the child for clues such as a PEFR meter, inhalers, etc.

Table 24. Normal respiratory rates in children	
Age in years	**Respiratory rate (breaths per minute)**
Premature infant	40–60
Term infant	30–50
6 years	19–24
12 years	16–21

Look for:

- Deformities of the chest (barrel chest, *pectus excavatum*, *pectus carinatum*) and spine.
- Asymmetry of chest expansion.
- Signs of respiratory distress such as the use of accessory muscles of respiration, suprasternal, intercostal, and/or subcostal recession, nasal flaring, and difficulty speaking.
- Harrison's sulci.
- Operative scars.

Inspection and examination of the hands

- Take both hands and assess them for colour and temperature.
- Look for clubbing.
- Determine the rate, rhythm, and character of the radial pulse (in younger infants, the brachial pulse).
- State that you would record the blood pressure.

Inspection and examination of the head and neck

- Inspect the conjunctivae for signs of anaemia.
- Inspect the mouth for signs of central cyanosis.
- Assess the jugular venous pressure and jugular venous pulse form.
- Palpate the cervical, supraclavicular, infraclavicular, and axillary lymph nodes.

Palpation of the chest

 Ask the child if he has any pain in the chest.

- Palpate for tracheal deviation by placing the index and middle fingers of one hand on either side of the trachea in the suprasternal notch. (As this may be uncomfortable, it is probably best omitted in younger children.)
- Palpate for the position of the cardiac apex.

[Note]   Carry out all subsequent steps on the front of the chest and, once this is done, repeat them on the back of the chest.

- Palpate for equal chest expansion, comparing one side to the other.
- Palpate for tactile fremitus.

Percussion of the chest

- Percuss the chest. Start at the apex of one lung and compare one side to the other. Do not forget to percuss over the clavicles and on the sides of the chest. Note that percussion of the chest is not useful in young infants.

Auscultation of the chest

 Warm up the diaphragm of your stethoscope.

- If old enough, ask the child to take deep breaths through the mouth and, using the diaphragm of the stethoscope, auscultate the chest. Start at the apex of one lung, and compare one side to the other. Are the breath sounds vesicular or bronchial? Are there any added sounds?

After the examination

- Cover the child.
- Ask the child and parent if they have any questions or concerns.
- Thank the child and parent.
- Indicate that you would like to look at the sputum pot, measure the PEFR and, if appropriate, order some key investigations, e.g. a CXR, FBC, etc.
- Summarise your findings and offer a differential diagnosis.

Most common conditions likely to come up in a paediatric examination: respiratory system station
Asthma
Cystic fibrosis
Broncho-pulmonary dysplasia
Pneumonia

Station 59

Paediatric examination: abdomen

Before starting

- Introduce yourself to the child and parent.
- Explain the examination and ask for consent to carry it out.
- Position the child so that he is lying flat and expose his abdomen as much as possible (customarily 'nipples to knees', although this is not appropriate in an OSCE setting).
- Ensure that he is comfortable.

The examination

General inspection

- From the end of the couch, observe the child's general appearance:
  - does the child look his age? Ask to look at the growth chart
  - nutritional status
  - state of health/other obvious signs
- Inspect the abdomen noting any:
  - distension
  - localised masses
  - scars and skin changes
- Look around the child for clues such as oxygen, tubes, drains, etc.

 A distended abdomen is often a normal finding in younger infants.

Inspection and examination of the hands

- Take both hands looking for:
  - temperature and colour
  - clubbing
  - nail signs
- Take the pulse.

Inspection and examination of the head, neck, and upper body

- Inspect the sclera and conjunctivae for signs of jaundice or anaemia.
- Inspect the mouth, looking for ulcers (Crohn's disease), angular stomatitis (nutritional deficiency), atrophic glossitis (iron deficiency, vitamin B12 deficiency, folate deficiency), furring of the tongue (loss of appetite), and the state of the dentition.
- Examine the neck for lymphadenopathy.

Palpation of the abdomen

- Abdominal palpation can be difficult in children if they do not relax the abdominal muscles. Attempt to distract the child by handing him a toy or try to make him relax by coaxing him into palpating his abdomen and then copying his actions.

 Ask the child if he has any tummy pain and keep your eyes on his face as you begin palpating his abdomen.

- *Light palpation* – begin by palpating furthest from the area of pain or discomfort and systematically palpate in the four quadrants and the umbilical area. Look for tenderness, guarding, and any masses.
- *Deep palpation* – for greater precision. Describe and localise any masses.

Palpation of the organs

- *Liver* – starting in the right lower quadrant, feel for the liver edge using the flat of your hand. Note that in younger infants the liver edge is normally palpable.
- *Spleen* – palpate for the spleen as for the liver, starting in the right lower quadrant.
- *Kidneys* – position the child close to the edge of the bed and ballot each kidney using the technique of deep bimanual palpation. Beyond the neonatal period, it is unlikely that you should be able to feel a normal kidney.

Percussion

- Percuss the liver area, also remembering to detect its upper border.
- Percuss the suprapubic area for dullness (bladder distension).
- If the abdomen is distended, test for shifting dullness (ascites).

Auscultation

- Auscultate in the mid-abdomen for abdominal sounds. Listen for 30 seconds at least before concluding that they are hyperactive, hypoactive, or absent.

Examination of the groins and genitalia

- Inspect the groins for hernias and, in boys, examine the testes (this is particularly important in younger infants).
- Note that examination of the groins and genitalia may only need to be mentioned, as it is not usually carried out in the OSCE setting.

Rectal examination

- PR is not routine practice in paediatrics and should be avoided unless specifically indicated.

After the examination

- Ask to test the urine.
- Cover the child.
- Ask the child and parent if they have any questions or concerns.
- Indicate that you would test the urine and order some key investigations, e.g. ultrasound scan, FBC, LFTs, U&Es, and clotting screen.
- Thank the child and parent.
- Summarise your findings and offer a differential diagnosis.

Most common conditions likely to come up in a paediatric examination: abdomen station
Constipation
Coeliac disease
Kidney transplant

Station 60

Paediatric examination: gait and neurological function

Before starting

- Introduce yourself to the child and parent.
- Tell the child that you are going to examine him.
- Ensure that he is comfortable.

 Examination of neurological function in children is principally a matter of observation. If the child is old enough to obey commands, a more formal assessment of gait and neurological function can be carried out, as in adults.

The examination

Neurological overview

- A brief developmental assessment should be performed to enable you to gauge the child's subsequent performance. Ask the parent the child's age and if there are any concerns about the child's vision and/or hearing.

Gait and movement

- If the child is too young to walk, observe him crawling or playing. Is he using all his limbs equally?
- If possible, observe the child walking and running. Common abnormalities of gait in children include:
  - scissoring or tiptoeing gait – suggestive of cerebral palsy or of Duchenne muscular dystrophy
  - broad-based gait: suggestive of a cerebellar disorder
  - limp – limps have many causes including dislocated hip, trauma, sepsis, and arthritis
- If possible, observe the child rising from the floor. The Gower sign (the child rising from the floor by 'climbing' up his legs) is suggestive of Duchenne muscular dystrophy.

Inspection

- Inspect all four limbs, in particular looking for muscle wasting or hypertrophy. Hypertrophy of the calves is suggestive of Duchenne muscular dystrophy.

Tone

- Assess tone and range of movement in all four limbs.
- In younger children also assess truncal tone by trying to get the child to sit unsupported.
- In young infants test head lag by lying the infant supine and pulling up his upper body by the arms.

Power

- Observe the child playing, and look for appropriate anti-gravity movement. A more formal assessment can be carried out if the child is old enough to carry out instructions.

Reflexes

- Check all reflexes as in the adult. Practice is the key!
- Note that eliciting the Babinsky sign (extensor plantar reflex) is not very discriminative in children.

Co-ordination

- If the child is old enough to carry out instructions, assess co-ordination by the finger-to-nose test or just by asking the child to jump or hop. If the child cannot carry out instructions, give him toys or some bricks and assess his co-ordination by observing him at play.

Sensation

- Indicate that you would test sensation.

Cranial nerves

- Indicate that you would test the cranial nerves – where possible this is done as in the adult.

After the examination

- Thank the parent and child.
- If appropriate, indicate that you would order some key investigations, e.g. CT, MRI, nerve conduction studies, electromyography, etc.
- Summarise your findings and offer a differential diagnosis.

Most common conditions likely to come up in a paediatric examination: gait and neurological function station
Ex-premature infant
Cerebral palsy
Duchenne muscular dystrophy
Myotonic dystrophy

Infant and child Basic Life Support

Specifications: A mannequin in lieu of an infant or child.

[Note]   For the purposes of Basic Life Support, an infant is defined as being under 1 year, and a child as being between 1 year and puberty.

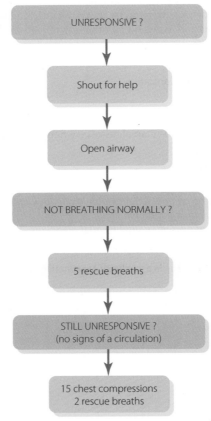

UNRESPONSIVE ?

Shout for help

Open airway

NOT BREATHING NORMALLY ?

5 rescue breaths

STILL UNRESPONSIVE ?
(no signs of a circulation)

15 chest compressions
2 rescue breaths

After 1 minute call resuscitation team then continue CPR

Figure 45. Paediatric Basic Life Support algorithm.

- Ensure the safety of the rescuer and child
- Check the child's responsiveness by gently stimulating the child and asking loudly, 'Are you all right?'

Do not shake infants or children with suspected cervical spine injuries.

- If the child responds by answering or moving:
  - leave the child in the position in which you find him (provided he is not in further danger)
  - check his condition and get help if needed

- reassess him regularly
- If the child does not respond:
  - shout for help
  - open the child's airway by using the head-tilt, chin-lift technique (see *Station 86*); if you have difficulty opening the airway using the head-tilt, chin-lift technique, try the jaw-thrust technique (see *Station 87*) – both methods may be easier to carry out if the child is turned onto his back

 If you suspect that there may have been injury to the neck, try to open the airway using chin lift or jaw thrust alone. If this is unsuccessful, add head tilt a small amount at a time until the airway is open.

- Holding the child's airway open, put your face close to his mouth and look along his chest. Listen, feel, and look for breathing for no more than 10 seconds.
- If the child is breathing normally:
  - turn him into the recovery position
  - check for continued breathing
- If he is not breathing normally or is making agonal gasps (infrequent, irregular breaths):
  - carefully remove any obvious airway obstruction
  - give 5 initial rescue breaths
- While performing the rescue breaths, note any gag or cough response to your action.
- To deliver rescue breaths to a child over 1 year:
  - ensure head tilt and chin lift
  - pinch the soft part of his nose closed with the index finger and thumb of the hand on his forehead
  - allow his mouth to open, but maintain chin lift
  - take a breath and place your lips around his mouth, making sure that you have a good seal
  - blow steadily into his mouth over 1–1.5 seconds, watching for his chest to rise
  - maintaining head tilt and chin lift, take your mouth away from the victim and watch for his chest to fall
  - take another breath and repeat this sequence 5 times
- To deliver rescue breaths to an infant:
  - ensure a neutral position of the head and apply chin lift
  - take a breath and cover the mouth and nasal apertures of the infant with your mouth, making sure you have a good seal
  - blow steadily into the infant's mouth and nose over 1–1.5 seconds so that the chest rises visibly
  - maintaining head tilt and chin lift, take your mouth away from the victim and watch for his chest to fall
  - take another breath and repeat this sequence 5 times
- If you have difficulty achieving an effective breath, the airway may be obstructed.
  - Open the child's mouth and remove any visible obstruction.
  - Ensure that there is adequate head tilt and chin lift, but also that the neck is not over extended.
  - If the head-tilt, chin-lift method has not opened the airway, try the jaw thrust method.
  - Make 5 attempts to achieve effective rescue breaths. If still unsuccessful, move on to chest compression.
- Check for signs of a circulation (signs of life).
- Take no more than 10 seconds to check for signs of circulation such as movement, coughing, or normal breathing (but not agonal gasps).

- Check the pulse but take no longer than 10 seconds to do this. In a child check the carotid pulse, in an infant check the brachial pulse.
- If you are confident that you have detected signs of circulation:
  - continue rescue breathing, if necessary, until the child starts breathing effectively on his own
  - turn the child into the recovery position if he remains unconscious
  - reassess the child frequently
- If there are no signs of a circulation,
  - *or* no pulse,
  - *or* a slow pulse (less than 60 per minute with poor perfusion),
  - *or* you are not sure,
- start chest compression. To deliver chest compressions to all children, compress the lower third of the sternum.
  - Locate the xiphisternum and compress the sternum one finger's breadth above this.
  - Compress the sternum by approximately one-third of the depth of the chest. In infants, use the tips of two fingers or, if there are two or more rescuers, use the encircling technique with two thumbs. In children, use the heel of one hand or, in larger children, the heels of both hands, as in adults.
  - Aim for a rate of 100 compressions per minute.
- After 15 compressions, tilt the head, lift the chin, and give two effective breaths.
- Continue compressions and breaths in a ratio of 15:2 (lone rescuers may use a ratio of 30:2).
- Continue resuscitation until the child shows signs of life (spontaneous respiration, pulse, movement) or further help arrives or you become exhausted.

When to go for assistance

- If more than one rescuer is present, one rescuer begins resuscitation whilst another goes for assistance.
- If only one rescuer is present, he should undertake resuscitation for 1 minute before going for assistance. It may be possible for him to carry the infant or child whilst going for assistance.
- The exception to this rule is in the case of a child with a witnessed, sudden collapse when the rescuer is alone. In this case the cause is likely to be an arrhythmia and the child may need defibrillation. Go for assistance immediately if there is no one to go for you.

Adapted from Resuscitation Council (UK), 2005 Guidelines.

Child immunisation programme

The instructions for this station may involve explaining the immunisation programme to a parent, or talking to an anxious parent about the pros and cons of the MMR vaccine. This station covers the facts, see *Station 110: Explaining skills* for the method.

Table 25. The UK Immunisation schedule

Age	Vaccine	Specifications
Birth	BCG	If at risk of tuberculosis
2 months	DTP triple vaccine • diphtheria • tetanus • pertussis Hib Polio	One injection
	Meningococcus type C	One injection
3 months	As for 2 months	
4 months	As for 2 months	
12–15 months	MMR • measles • mumps • rubella	One injection
3½ years (preschool age)	Diphtheria Tetanus Pertussis Polio MMR	Boosters
10–14 years	BCG	If indicated by Heaf testing
16 years (school leavers)	Diphtheria Tetanus Polio	Boosters

The MMR controversy

- Measles can cause pneumonia, fits, encephalitis, sub-acute sclerosing panencephalitis, and death.
- Mumps can cause meningitis, encephalitis, deafness, and sterility.
- Rubella in pregnancy can cause severe damage to the foetus.
- The MMR vaccine is safe and effective, and more than 500 million doses of the vaccine have been given since 1972.
- Common side-effects of the MMR vaccine are a sore injection site and flu-like symptoms. Very rarely, an allergic reaction can occur.
- There is no evidence to support a distinct syndrome of MMR-induced autism or inflammatory bowel disease.
- Separate administration of the measles, mumps, and rubella vaccines provides no added benefit over administration of the combined MMR vaccine, but means three injections and potentially delayed or missed vaccinations.

Geriatric history

Before starting

- Introduce yourself to the patient.
- Explain that you are going to ask him some questions to determine the nature of his problems, and ask for his consent to do this.
- Ensure that he is comfortable; if not, make sure that he is.
- Ask if you can take a collateral history from a caretaker.

The history

- Name, age, and past occupation if this information has not already been provided.

Presenting complaint

- Enquire about the presenting complaint, if any. Use open questions and active listening.
- Elicit the patient's ideas, concerns, and expectations.
- Enquire about the effects that his symptoms are having on his life.

Then aim to cover:

- Physical independence, e.g. describe a typical day.
- Functional assessment: can he stand up and walk, climb the stairs, get on and off the toilet, get in and out of the bathtub, dress, cook/clean/shop, and manage his finances and administration?
- Living arrangements: housing, heating, lighting, stairs, toileting, slippery bathtubs, loose rugs, cooker and smoke alarm, adaptive or home safety aids, e.g. grab bars in the bathroom, stair lift, raised toilet seat, shower stool, bedside commode, etc.
- Carers and support services.
- Social interaction: family, friends, clubs, etc. If appropriate, ask *"Who will help you if you become ill? Who should make decisions for you if you become too ill to speak for yourself?"*
- Daily diet, including nausea, vomiting, and change in appetite or weight.
- Mood (e.g. *"How are you keeping in your spirits?"*). Also ask about sleep and appetite.
- Memory and cognitive impairment.
- Dizziness/falls (see *Station 30: History of 'funny turns'*).
- Vision (corrective aids, accidents, difficulty reading, feeding, dressing, grooming, driving, and recognising pills or items).
- Urinary and faecal incontinence.
- Smoking and alcohol use.

Past medical history

- Current, past, and childhood illnesses. Ask about rheumatic fever and polio.
- Surgery.

Drug history

- Prescribed medication and *compliance*.
- Over-the-counter drugs.
- Allergies.

Family history

- Parents, siblings, and children. Ask specifically about diabetes, Alzheimer's disease, and cancer.

After taking the history

- Ask the patient if there is anything that he might add that you have forgotten to ask about.
- Ask if he has any questions or concerns.
- Thank him.
- Indicate that you would like to examine the patient and order some investigations.
- Formulate a problem list and suggest treatment options.

Station 64

Geriatric physical examination

Examining a patient in old age (>65 years old) is very similar to examining a patient at any other age. If asked to examine a patient in old age, important features to look out for or aspects to consider are:

Vital signs

Temperature, pulse, blood pressure (lying and standing), respiratory rate, height, weight.

General inspection

Nutritional status, posture, tremor, gait, aids

Skin

Pressure sores, senile keratoses, senile purpura, bruises, pre-malignant or malignant lesions.

Eyes, ears, nose and throat

Vision (including fundoscopy), hearing, mouth, throat.

Musculoskeletal system

Arthritis, muscle wasting, contractures, range of motion in different joints.

Cardiovascular system

Arrhythmias, added sounds, murmurs, carotid bruits, pedal oedema, absent peripheral pulses, gangrene.

Respiratory system

Chest expansion, basal crackles (may be difficult to hear because of basilar rales).

Abdomen

Organomegaly, bladder distension, abdominal aortic aneurysm, frequency and quality of abdominal sounds, rectal examination.

Breast and genitourinary

Malignancy.

Neurological examination

Tone, power, sensation, reflexes, gait, co-ordination.

Figure 46. Senile purpura.

© Dermatlas; www.dermatlas.org – reproduced with permission.

Obstetric history

Specifications: You may be asked to focus on only a certain aspect or certain aspects of the obstetric history.

Before starting

- Introduce yourself to the patient.
- Explain that you are going to ask her some questions to uncover the nature and background of her obstetric complaint, and ask for consent to do this.
- Ensure that she is comfortable.

The history

- Name, age, and occupation.

Presenting problem (presenting complaint)

Ask about the presenting problem (if any) in some detail.

History of the present pregnancy

- Determine the duration of gestation and calculate the expected due date (EDD).
  - Ask about the date of the patient's last menstrual period (LMP).
  - Ask if her periods had been regular prior to her LMP.
  - Ask if she had been on the oral contraceptive pill (OCP). If yes, determine when she stopped taking it and the number of periods she had before becoming pregnant.
  - Determine the duration of gestation and calculate the EDD. To calculate the EDD add 9 months and 7 days to the date of the LMP. If this proves too arduous a task, try adding one year, subtracting three months, and adding 7 days.
- Ask about foetal movements and, if present, about any changes in their frequency.
- Take a detailed history of the pregnancy, enquiring about:

First trimester:

  - date and method of pregnancy confirmation
  - was the pregnancy planned or unplanned? If it was unplanned, is it desired?
  - symptoms of pregnancy (e.g. sickness, indigestion, headaches, dizziness…)
  - bleeding during pregnancy
  - ultrasound scan (10–12/52)
  - chorionic villus sampling (10–13/52)
  - type of antenatal care (e.g. shared care, midwife-led care, domino scheme, consultant-led scheme)

Second trimester:

  - amniocentesis (16–18/52)
  - anomaly scan (18–20/52)
  - quickening (16–18/52)

Third trimester:

  - antenatal clinic findings – you *must* ask about blood pressure and proteinuria

- vaginal bleeding
- hospital admissions

History of previous pregnancies (past reproductive history)

Ask her if she has any children.

For each previous pregnancy, ask about:

The pregnancy, including:

- the date (year) of birth
- the duration of the pregnancy and any problems
- the mode of delivery and any problems
- the outcome

The child, including:

- the child's birth weight
- problems after birth
- the child's present condition

 Do not forget to also ask about miscarriages, stillbirths, and terminations.

Gynaecological history

Take a focussed gynaecological history, and ask about the date and result of the last cervical smear test.

Past medical history

- Current, past, and childhood illnesses.
- Surgery.
- Recent visits to the doctor.

Drug history

- Prescribed medication.
- Over-the-counter drugs.
- Smoking.
- Alcohol use.
- Recreational drug use.
- Allergies.

Family history

- Parents, siblings, and children. Has anyone in the family ever had a similar problem?
- Is there a family history of hypertension, heart disease, or diabetes?
- *Is there a history of twins or triplets in your family or in your partner's family?*

Social history

- Support from the partner and/or family.
- Employment.
- Income and financial support.
- Housing.

After taking the history

- Ask the patient if there is anything she might add that you have forgotten to ask about.
- Thank the patient.
- If asked, summarise your findings and offer a differential diagnosis.

Examination of the pregnant woman

Specifications: Most likely an anatomical model in lieu of a patient.

Before examining the patient

- Introduce yourself to the patient.
- Explain the examination and ensure consent.
- Indicate that you would weigh the patient, take her blood pressure (pre-eclampsia), dipstick her urine (pre-eclampsia, gestational diabetes) and ask her to empty her bladder.
- Position the patient so that she is lying supine (she can sit up if she finds lying supine uncomfortable).
- Ask her to expose her abdomen.
- Ensure that she is comfortable.

The examination

General inspection

Carry out a general inspection from the end of the couch.

Inspection of the abdomen

- Abdominal distension and symmetry.
- *Linea nigra.*
- *Striae gravidarum.*
- Scars.

Palpation of the abdomen

Facing the mother, determine the:

- size of the uterus
- liquor volume (normal, polyhydramnios, oligohydramnios)
- number of foetuses
- size of the foetus(es)
- lie
- presenting part

Turning to face the mother's feet, determine the:

- engagement

Table 26. Some important obstetric definitions

Lie. The relationship of the long axis of the foetus to that of the uterus, described as longitudinal, transverse, or oblique.

Presenting part. The part of the foetus that is in relation with the pelvic inlet, e.g. cephalic/breech for a longitudinal lie or shoulder/arm for a transverse/oblique lie.

Engagement. During engagement, the presenting part descends into the pelvic inlet in readiness for labour. Engagement is usually described in fifths of head palpable above the pelvic inlet, although sometimes the presenting part may not be the head. Prior to engagement, the foetus is said to be 'floating' or ballotable.

Although not usually performed, indicate that you could also determine the position, station, and attitude of the foetus. Position refers to the relationship of a point of reference on the foetus to the quadranted pelvis; station refers to the depth of the presenting part in relation to the ischial spines (from −5 to +5); attitude refers to the degree of flexion of the foetus' body parts.

Symphyseal–fundal height (SFH)

Using a tape measure, measure from the mid-point of the symphysis pubis to the top of the uterus. From 20 to 38 weeks of gestation, the SFH in centimetres approximates to the number of weeks of gestation ± 2.

Auscultation

Listen to the foetal heart by placing a Pinard stethoscope over the foetus' anterior shoulder and estimate the heart rate (usually 110–160 bpm). Ensure that your hands are free from the abdomen.

After the examination

- Cover the patient up.
- Thank the patient.
- Summarise your findings.

Gynaecological history

Specifications: You may be asked to circumscribe your questioning to certain aspects of the gynaecological history only.

Before starting

- Introduce yourself to the patient.
- Explain that you are going to ask her some questions to uncover the nature and background of her gynaecological complaint, and ask for her consent to do this.
- Ensure that she is comfortable.

The history

- Name, age, and occupation.

Presenting complaint and history of presenting complaint

- Enquire in detail about the nature of the presenting complaint and the history of the presenting complaint. First listen to the patient. Then ask about:
  - age at menarche
  - regularity of the menses
  - dysmenorrhoea
  - date of LMP – did the LMP seem normal?
  - vaginal discharge – if there is a vaginal discharge, ask about its amount, colour, and smell. Is it causing the patient to itch?
  - date and result of the last cervical smear test
  - vaginal prolapse
  - urinary incontinence
  - coitus, present or past (*"Are you sexually active?"*)
  - dyspareunia
  - use of contraception

Past medical history

- Past gynaecological history.
- Past reproductive history: previous pregnancies in chronological order, including terminations and miscarriages.
- Past medical history:
  - current, past, and childhood illnesses
  - surgery
  - recent visits to the doctor

Drug history

  - Prescribed medication.
  - Over-the-counter medication.
  - Recreational drug use.
  - Allergies.

Family history

- Ask about parents, siblings, children. Has anyone in the family had a similar problem? In the case of a suspected STD, don't forget to ask about the partner.

Social history

- Employment.
- Housing and home-help.
- Travel.
- Smoking.
- Alcohol use.

After taking the history

- Ask the patient if there is anything she might add that you have forgotten to ask about.
- Thank the patient.
- Summarise your findings and offer a differential diagnosis.

Gynaecological (bimanual) examination

Specifications: A pelvic model in lieu of a patient.

Before starting

- Introduce yourself to the patient.
- Explain the examination, reassuring the patient that, although it may feel uncomfortable, it should not cause any pain.
- Obtain consent.
- Ask for a chaperone.
- Confirm that the patient has emptied her bladder.
- Indicate that you would normally carry out an abdominal examination prior to a gynaecological examination.
- Once undressed, ask the patient to lie flat on the couch, bringing her heels to her buttocks and then letting her knees flop out.
- Ensure that she is comfortable, and cover her up with a drape.

The examination

 Always tell the patient what you are about to do.

- Don a pair of non-sterile gloves.
- Inspect the vulva, paying close attention to:
    - the pattern of hair distribution
    - the labia majora
    - the clitoris
- Palpate the labia majora.
- Try to palpate Bartholin's gland (the structure is not normally palpable).
- Lubricate the index and middle fingers of your gloved right hand.
- Use the thumb and index finger of your left hand to separate the labia minora.
- Insert the index and middle fingers of your right hand into the vagina at an angle of 45 degrees.
- Palpate the vaginal walls.
- Use your fingertips to palpate the cervix. Assess the cervix for size, shape, consistency, and mobility. Is the cervix tender? Is it open?
- Palpate the uterus: place the palmar surface of your left hand about 5 cm above the symphysis pubis and the internal fingers of your right hand behind the cervix and gently try to appose your fingers in an attempt to 'catch' the uterus. Assess the uterus for size, position, consistency, mobility, and tenderness. Can you feel any masses?

Figure 47. Technique for bimanual examination

- Palpate the right adnexae: place the palmar surface of your left hand in the right iliac fossa and the internal fingers of your right hand in the right fornix and gently try to appose your fingers in an attempt to 'catch' the ovary. Can you elicit excitation tenderness? (Look at the patient's face.)
- Use a similar technique for palpating the left adnexae.
- Once you have removed your internal fingers, inspect the glove for any blood or discharge.

After the examination

- Indicate that you could also have carried out a speculum examination and taken a cervical smear (see *Station 69: Cervical smear test*).
- Offer the patient a box of tissues and give her the opportunity to dress.
- Thank the patient.
- Ensure that she is comfortable.
- Summarise your findings and offer a differential diagnosis.

Most common conditions likely to come up in a gynaecological examination station
Uterine fibroids
Ovarian cyst

Cervical smear test and liquid based cytology test

Specifications: An anatomical model in lieu of a patient.

Before starting

- Introduce yourself to the patient.
- Explain the procedure to her, and ask her for her consent to carry it out.
- Request a chaperone.
- Confirm that the patient has emptied her bladder.
- Once undressed, ask the patient to lie flat on the couch, bringing her heels to her buttocks and then letting her knees flop out.
- Ensure that she is comfortable, and cover her up with a drape.
- Gather the appropriate equipment.

The equipment

On a trolley, gather:

- non-sterile gloves
- Ayres spatula
- fixative spray (or 95% alcohol)

- bivalve speculum
- brush, if post-menopausal
- labelled slides (name, date of birth, hospital number)

The procedure

- Indicate that you would record the patient's name, date of birth, and hospital number on the slide.
- Adjust the light source to ensure maximum visibility.
- Don the pair of gloves.
- Warm the speculum's blades in your palm.
- Place a small amount of K-Y jelly on either side of the speculum near the tip.
- With your non-dominant hand, part the labia to ensure all hair and skin are out of the way.
- With your other hand, slowly but gently, insert the speculum with the screw facing sideways, rotating it into position (screw upwards) and then opening it.
- Place the back of your non-dominant hand against her pubic area and gently open the speculum to identify the cervix.
- Fix the speculum in the open position by tightening the screw.

 A smear should not be taken if there is any bleeding or vaginal discharge.

- Place the tip of the Ayres spatula in the external os and rotate the spatula by 360 degrees in either direction, all the while keeping it firmly applied to the cervix.
- Spread the material thus obtained evenly onto the labelled slides.
- Immediately spray fixative onto the slides.
- Carefully remove the speculum. Hold the speculum in the open position and completely unscrew it. Then remove the speculum slowly allowing it to close naturally as you withdraw it.

Ayres spatula

Bladder

Uterus

Cervix

Figure 48. The cervical smear test.

After the procedure

- Dispose of the speculum and of the gloves.
- Offer the patient a box of tissues and give her the opportunity to dress.
- Warn her about the possibility of spotting/bleeding after the test.
- Explain to her when and how she will receive the test results, the possible outcomes, and when her next screening test is (i.e. 3 yearly if between 25 and 49 years of age, or 5 yearly if between 50 and 64 years of age).
- Ask the patient if she has any questions or concerns.
- Thank the patient.

Liquid based cytology test

Liquid based cytology (LBC) is a new method of preparing cervical samples for examination in the laboratory. It is currently being introduced and is soon to replace the conventional cervical smear test. If asked to perform an LBC test you must gather a pair of non-sterile gloves, a cervical examination brush (Cervex-Brush®), a vial containing preservative fluid, a bivalve speculum, and some K-Y jelly. Then you must carry out the following steps, the first four of which are similar to those outlined above:

- Check the expiry date on the sample collection vial and record the patient's name, date of birth and hospital number on both the vial and cytology request form.
- Adjust the light source.
- Don the pair of gloves.
- Warm, lubricate, and insert the speculum (see above).
- Insert the central bristles of the cervical brush into the endocervical canal and rotate it by 360 degrees in a clockwise direction five times.
- Immediately rinse the cervical brush in the preservative fluid by pushing it into the bottom of the vial ten times, forcing the bristles apart. Then swirl the brush vigorously to further release material.
- Inspect the cervical brush to ensure that it is free of material.
- Discard the brush.
- Carefully remove the speculum (see above).
- Tighten the cap on the vial and place it in a specimen bag, along with the request form.

Examiner's questions

Staging of cervical cancer:

Stages are described in terms of the International Federation of Gynecology and Obstetrics (FIGO) system, which is based on clinical rather than surgical findings.

Stage 0   Carcinoma *in situ*. Tumour is present only in epithelium.

Stage I   Invasive cancer with tumour strictly confined to cervix.

Stage II   Invasive cancer with tumour extending beyond cervix or upper two-thirds of vagina, but not onto pelvic wall.

Stage III   Invasive cancer with tumour spreading to lower third of vagina or onto pelvic wall.

Stage IV   Invasive cancer with tumour spreading to other parts of the body.

NB: Various sub-stages are also described.

Station 70

Breast history

Before starting

- Introduce yourself to the patient.
- Explain that you are going to ask her some questions to uncover the nature of her complaint, and ask for her consent to do this.
- Ensure that she comfortable; if not, ensure that she is.

The history

- Name, age, and occupation, if this information has not already been provided. Is the patient pregnant or lactating?

Presenting complaint and history of presenting complaint

- Use open questions to ask about the presenting complaint.
- Ask specifically about pain, a lump in the breast, and nipple discharge.

For pain, determine:

- Site.
- Severity.
- Nature.
- Onset.
- Duration.
- Aggravating and alleviating factors.
- Associated signs and symptoms:
  - locally, e.g. lump, discharge, bleeding, skin changes, nipple retraction/inversion
  - systemically, e.g. tiredness, fever, night sweats, weight loss, chest or back pain
- Cyclicity.
- If the patient has had it before.
- Any other changes in the breast.

For a lump in the breast, determine:

- Site.
- Size.
- Onset.
- Duration.
- Cyclicity.
- Associated symptoms:
  - locally, e.g. pain, discharge, bleeding, skin changes, nipple retraction/inversion
  - systemically, e.g. tiredness, fever, night sweats, weight loss, chest or back pain
- If the patient has had it before.

For nipple discharge, determine:

- Amount.
- Colour.
- If it is unilateral or bilateral.
- If it is from one duct or several.
- If it is spontaneous.

- Associated symptoms:
  - locally, e.g. pain, lump, bleeding, skin changes, nipple retraction/inversion
  - systemically, e.g. tiredness, fever, night sweats, weight loss, chest or back pain
- If the patient has been breast-feeding.
- If the patient has had it before.

Past medical history

- Age at menarche and (if applicable) menopause. Does the patient have any children? How old are they? Did she breast-feed them?
- Current, past, and childhood illnesses.
- Surgery.
- Previous breast investigations.
- Recent visits to the doctor.

Drug history

- Prescribed medication, especially oral contraceptives and HRT. Note that certain drugs, e.g. antipsychotics, can cause hyperprolactinaemia and galactorrhoea.
- Over-the-counter medications.
- Recreational drug use.
- Allergies.

Family history

- Parents, siblings, and children. Ask specifically about breast problems and cancers.

Social history

- Smoking.
- Alcohol use.
- Employment, past and present.
- Housing.
- Hobbies.

Systems enquiry

(If appropriate.)

After taking the history

- Ask the patient if there is anything that she might add that you have forgotten to ask about.
- Thank the patient.
- Summarise your findings and offer a differential diagnosis.
- State that you would like to examine the patient and possibly order some investigations, e.g. mammogram, ultrasound scan, fine-needle aspiration cytology (FNAC), to confirm your diagnosis.

Most common conditions likely to come up in breast history station	
Fibroadenoma	Mammary duct ectasia
Fibrocystic disease	Carcinoma
Mastitis	Intraductal papilloma
Breast abscess	

Breast examination

Specifications: In this station you may be asked to examine a patient wearing synthetic breasts. You may also be asked to take a brief history beforehand.

A full breast examination involves inspection, palpation of the breast tissue, palpation of the nipple, and palpation of the lymph nodes.

Before starting

- Introduce yourself to the patient.
- Explain the examination, and ask her for consent to carry it out.
- Request a chaperone.
- Ask her to undress from the waist up and hand her a drape or blanket to cover herself up with.
- Ask her to sit on the edge of the couch, and ensure that she is comfortable.

The examination

General inspection

- From a distance, observe the patient's general appearance (age, state of health, any obvious signs).

Inspection of the breasts

- Note the size, symmetry, contour, and colour of the breast; also note the pattern of venous drainage. In particular, look for the important signs of nipple inversion or retraction and *peau d'orange* (breast carcinoma). Is there a visible discharge? Are there any scars? Also remember to look under the breasts (ask the patient to lift up her breasts for you).
- Now ask the patient to put her hands atop her head and then to press them against her hips. Look for tethering and asymmetrical changes in the breast contour.

Palpation of the breasts

- Ask the patient to sit back on the couch, reclining at 45 degrees.
- Warm up your hands.
- Before palpating the breasts, ask if there is any breast or chest pain.
- Starting with the normal breast, palpate the breast tissue with the palmar surface of the middle three fingers, using an even rotary movement to compress the breast tissue gently towards the chest wall. If the breasts are large, use one hand to steady the breast on its lower border.
- Examine each breast following a concentric trail.

Directions of palpation over breast surface

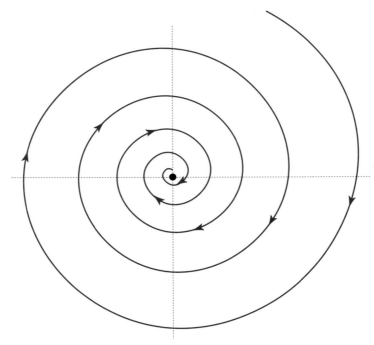

Figure 49. The circular palpation technique. Other palpation techniques include the vertical strip and wedge techniques.

- Ask the patient to put her hands atop her head and palpate the tail of Spence between thumb and forefinger.

Assess any lump for size, shape, consistency, mobility, surface, temperature, and tenderness.

 Don't forget that there are two breasts that need examining, a common enough oversight in the artificial and anxiety-provoking OSCE situation.

Palpation of the nipple

- Hold the nipple between thumb and forefinger and gently compress it in an attempt to express a discharge (or ask the patient to do this). A discharge could signify normal lactation, galactorrhoea, duct ectasia, a carcinoma, or an intraductal papilloma. Any fluid expressed should be smeared for cytology and swabbed for microbiology.

Palpation of the lymph nodes

- Expose the right axilla by lifting and abducting the arm and supporting it at the wrist with your right hand.
- With your left hand, palpate the following lymph node groups (See *Figure 4*, p. 18):
  - apical
  - anterior
  - posterior

- infraclavicular and supraclavicular
- nodes of the medial aspect of the humerus
- Now expose the left axilla by lifting and abducting the left arm and supporting at the wrist with your left hand.
- With your right hand, palpate the lymph node groups, as listed above.

 Assess any nodes for size, shape, consistency, mobility, and tenderness.

After the examination

Indicate that you could also:

- palpate the liver edge for an enlarged liver (liver metastases)
- palpate the spine for tenderness (spinal metastases)
- auscultate the lung bases (pleural effusions)

- Cover up the patient.
- Thank the patient.
- Ensure that she is comfortable.
- Summarise your findings and offer a differential diagnosis.
- Offer further investigations if appropriate, e.g. mammogram, USS, or FNAC

Most common conditions likely to come up in a breast examination station	
Benign breast changes	Fibrocystic disease
Fibroadenoma	Carcinoma
Fibroadenosis	

Sexual history

 This is a history that students often find difficult because of the highly personal nature of the questions involved. The trick is to remain formal and professional throughout, yet to exert tact and, if the patient becomes uncomfortable, a measure of restraint. The OSCE may ask you to focus on either risk assessment or sexual function. If the latter, do not forget that sexual dysfunction often results from medical and psychiatric disorders and/ or their treatments, e.g. antihypertensives, antidepressants.

Before starting

- Introduce yourself to the patient.
- Set the scene: *"I'd like to ask you a few questions about your sex life. I don't mean to embarrass you, and it's alright if you prefer not to answer some of my questions. May I begin?"*
- Reassure the patient about confidentiality.

The history

Would you describe yourself as heterosexual, homosexual, or bisexual?

Who

- *"Who did you last have sex with, and when was this?"*
- *"Who else have you had sex with in the last three months?"*
- *"Were they regular or casual partners?"*
- *"Were they male or female (or both)?"*

How

- *"Did you have vaginal/oral/anal sex?"*
- *"If oral or anal sex, did you give it or receive it?"*
- *"Did you use protection on each occasion?"*
- If yes, *"did you have any problems with it?"*
- *"Have you ever been hurt or abused by your partner?"*

Where

- *"Have you had sex whilst abroad? Whom with?"*
- *"Where are your partners from?"*
- *"Is it possible that they have had sex whilst abroad?"*

Sexually transmitted diseases

Ask about:

- Any sores, discharge, itching, dysuria, and abdominal pain (in females). Explore any positive findings.
- History of sexually transmitted diseases (including HIV) in both the patient and his partner(s).
- In females, date and result of the last cervical smear test.

Sexual function

- *"Do you have any problems with, or concerns about, having sex?"* You may ask specifically about erectile dysfunction and ejaculatory dysfunction in males, and about hypoactive sexual desire, anorgasmia, vaginismus, and dyspareunia in females.
- Determine the onset, course, and duration of the problem. Is the problem primary or secondary?
- Determine the frequency and timing of the problem. Is the problem partial or situational? In situational erectile dysfunction, the patient is still able to have morning erections.
- Determine the effect that the problem is having on the patient's life.

Past medical history

Drug history

Family history

Social history including smoking, alcohol, and recreational drugs

After taking the history

- Ask if there is anything that the patient would like to add which you may have forgotten to ask about.
- Thank the patient.
- Summarise your findings and offer a further course of action.

Station 73

HIV risk assessment

Before starting

- Introduce yourself to the patient.
- Explain that you are going to ask him some questions to determine his risk of having contracted HIV, and ask him for his consent to do this.
- Remember to be especially sensitive, tactful, and empathetic.

The risk assessment

- Explore the patient's reason for attendance.

Sexual behaviour

Establish:

- Whether the patient has sex with men, women, or both.
- Whether he has had unprotected anal, vaginal, or oral sex. If so, when, where, how often, and with how many different partners? Receptive anal intercourse is especially high risk.
- Whether he has recently contracted any sexually transmitted diseases.
- The HIV status and sexual practices of the patient's partners.

Illicit drug use

Establish:

- Whether the patient has been injecting himself. If so, has he been sharing needles?
- Whether any of his partners inject themselves.

Blood products and transfusions

Establish:

- Whether the patient is a haemophiliac.
- Whether he has received blood products or transfusions prior to about 1985.

Occupational risk

- Ask about the patient's occupation to determine if he poses an occupational risk.

After the risk assessment

- Ask the patient if there is anything that he might add that you have forgotten to ask about.
- Give him feedback on his HIV risk and, if appropriate, indicate a further course of action, e.g. an HIV test.
- Address his concerns.
- Thank him.

Condom explanation

Male and female condoms are barrier methods of contraception and prevent sperm from reaching the egg. They are very effective at preventing sexually transmitted infections but less effective than methods such as the pill in preventing pregnancy.

There are many different types of male condoms available on the market. These include plain-end or teat-end, shaped/ribbed or straight-sided, and lubricated (e.g. with inert silicone or nonoxynol-9 spermicide) condoms. Femidom is the only female condom available in the UK.

Spermicidal condoms are no longer recommended as evidence suggests that nanoxynol-9 may increase the risk of HIV and other sexually transmitted infections such as chlamydia and gonorrhoea.

Before starting

- Introduce yourself to the patient.
- Establish how much he already knows about using condoms. If correctly used, the male condom is 98% effective, and the female condom is 95% effective. Condoms also protect against STDs.

The equipment

- Two condoms.
- A model of a penis.
- An information booklet on condom use.

Explain the use of a condom

Explain that condom use should be discussed with the partner(s) and that the condom should be put on before any genital contact has taken place.

Explain/demonstrate to:

- check for the British Kite mark or equivalent symbol, a guarantee of quality
- check the expiry date
- carefully tear open the pack and remove the condom – do not use teeth or sharp nails
- position the condom on the tip of the erect penis
- squeeze out the air from the tip of the condom and gently roll it out to the base of the penis
- hold the condom at the base of the penis during penetration
- after intercourse, remove the condom ensuring that semen is not spilt
- dispose of the condom in the bin – condoms must never be re-used

Ask the patient to repeat the procedure.

Figure 50. British kite mark.

🛈 *Explain that condoms can occasionally tear and that, in this event, the patient and his partner should consult a GP or family planning clinic.*

Principal side-effects are due to latex allergy and spermicide sensitivity.

Principal contraindications are oil-based lubricants such as Vaseline, hormonal vaginal creams, and antifungal preparations (Canesten is safe to use).

After the explanation

- Ask if the patient has any questions or concerns. (He may ask you about other methods of contraception.)
- Tell him to return should he have any further questions.
- Give him an information booklet on condom use.

Combined oral contraceptive pill (COCP) explanation

Before starting

- Introduce yourself to the patient.
- Ask for her name and age.
- Confirm the reason for her attendance.
- Has she considered other methods of contraception?

Explaining the COCP – items to cover

Efficacy

99.9% if used correctly, 97% in practice.

 It is important to emphasise that the pill does not protect against STDs.

Principal benefits

- More regular periods, less blood loss, fewer period pains.
- Decreased risk of ovarian cancer and endometrial cancer.
- Acne often improves.

Principal risks

- Increased risk of deep vein thrombosis and pulmonary embolism.
- Increased risk of myocardial infarction.
- Increased risk of breast cancer and adenoma of the cervix.

Principal adverse effects

- Headache.
- Nausea.
- Dizziness.
- Hypertension.
- Breast tenderness.
- Weight gain.
- Depression.

Principal contraindications

Absolute

- Thrombophlebitis, thromboembolitic disorder, or history of thromboembolism.
- Stroke.
- Ischaemic heart disease.
- Liver disease.
- Kidney disease.

Station 75   Combined oral contraceptive pill (COCP) explanation

- History of breast cancer or other oestrogen-dependent cancers of the reproductive organs.
- Pregnancy.

Relative

- Uncontrolled hypertension.
- Migraine.
- Smoking (> 15 cigarettes a day and over the age of 35).
- Abnormal vaginal bleeding.
- Sickle cell disease.
- Breast-feeding.
- Family history of hyperlipidaemia, heart disease, or kidney disease.

 Remember to take a quick drug history, as many common drugs such as ampicillin or carbamazepine can alter the effectiveness of the pill.

How to take the pills

- Start taking the pill on the first Sunday after periods begin.
- Take one pill a day at the same time every day for either 21 or 28 days, depending on the number of pills in the pack.
- After finishing the 28-day pack, start another one immediately (the last seven pills in the 28-day pack are 'dummy pills').
- After finishing the 21-day pack, stop taking the pill for 7 days and then start another pack.
- Use barrier contraception during the first month on the pill.
- If you develop vomiting or diarrhoea, use barrier contraception until your next period.

Figure 51. A 28-day pack.

What if pills are missed

If one pill is missed:

- take a pill as soon as you can remember to do so
- take the next pill at the regular time
- use barrier contraception for 7 days

If two pills are missed:

- take two pills a day for 2 days
- use barrier contraception for 7 days

If three pills are missed:

- stop taking the pill and start on another pack in 7 days' time

Before finishing

- Summarise and check understanding.
- Hand out a leaflet on the COCP.
- Tell the patient to report any severe or unexpected symptoms.

Examiner's questions

Other forms of contraception

Combined hormonal contraceptives are also available as a skin patch, worn for 3 out of every 4 weeks.

Low-dose progestogen-only contraceptives such as the traditional progestogen-only pill (POP, 'mini-pill'), subdermal implants (e.g. Norplant), and intrauterine systems (e.g. Mirena) inconsistently inhibit ovulation but thicken the cervical mucus and reduce sperm penetration, and also make the endometrium unsuitable for implantation. Intermediate-dose progestogen-only contraceptives such as the Cerazette pill are much more reliable at inhibiting ovulation, and high-dose progestogen-only contraceptives such as the injectable Depo-Provera inhibit ovulation completely (in the case of Depo-Provera, for up to 3 months).

The POP is taken continuously without any breaks. Whereas the COCP can be taken within a window of 12 hours, the mini-pill has a much shorter window of 3 hours. Thus, whilst the efficacy of the mini-pill is similar to that of the COCP, it is more dependent on user compliance. The POP is not affected by broad-spectrum antibiotics, and can often be used when the COCP is contraindicated, e.g. in smokers above the age of 35. It is contraindicated in cardiovascular disease, liver disease, breast cancer, ovarian cysts, and migraine. Side-effects, if any, are generally mild and transient. There is a small increased risk of ectopic pregnancy and breast cancer. Unlike the COCP, the POP does not regulate menstruation and can lead to either irregular menstruation or amenorrhoea.

Emergency post-coital contraception comes either in the form of an intrauterine device (IUD) or an emergency contraceptive pill (ECP, 'morning-after pill') that, in contrast to medical abortion methods, act before implantation, either by postponing ovulation or by preventing implantation. The Levonelle brand contains levonorgestrel which is a progestogen hormone, and is licensed for use up to 72 hours after intercourse. There is an approximate 80% reduction in the risk of pregnancy, to about 1–2% (this compares to virtually 0% for the IUD). Generally speaking, the advantages of using the ECP outweigh any theoretical or proven risks, and harm to a foetus that has already implanted is thought to be very unlikely. Side-effects include nausea, vomiting, abdominal pain, fatigue, headache, and dizziness. The ECP should not be confused with the 'abortion pill' (high dose mifepristone, RU 486).

Pessaries and suppositories explanation

 Read in conjunction with Station 110: Explaining skills.

Like tablets, pessaries and suppositories are medication. Suppositories are for rectal use, common examples being pain-killers and steroids, whereas pessaries are for vaginal use, common examples being antibiotics and progesterone.

They are used if oral drugs cannot be given, for example, in the post-operative period or if the patient is vomiting, and if the site of action of the drug is the rectum or vagina, or near enough, for example, the colon or cervix.

In this station you may be asked to explain the use of a pessary and/or a suppository to a patient. Both scenarios have been described here.

Before starting

- Introduce yourself to the patient.
- Confirm her/his reason for attendance.
- Ask her/him if she/he has ever used a pessary or suppository before.

The explanation: items to cover

 Be sensitive to the psychological and sociocultural issues involved in placing a finger into the vagina or rectum, and be sympathetic and understanding.

Pessaries

- Pessaries are bullet-shaped medicines designed for easy insertion into the vagina using your fingers or an applicator. Your body temperature will slowly dissolve the pessary and release the medicine into your vagina.
- Wash and dry your hands.
- Remove the pessary and applicator (if supplied) from its foil or wrapper.
- If an applicator is supplied, push the pessary into the hole at its end.
- Lie down with your knees bent and legs apart.
- Carefully push the pessary high up into your vagina, pointed end first, using either your fingers or the applicator.
- If using an applicator, push the plunger to release the pessary and then remove the applicator.
- Wash your hands afterwards.
- The pessary may leak from your vagina, so it may be best to insert it before bedtime and to use a sanitary towel to avoid staining of the clothes.
- If you miss a dose, insert the pessary as soon as you remember, and then carry on as normal.
- Check the expiry date before using your pessary.
- Store in a cool, dry place and out of children's reach.
- Continue using your pessaries until the course is completed, even if this means inserting them during your monthly period.

Suppositories

- Suppositories are bullet-shaped medicines designed for easy insertion into the lower bowel (rectum) using your fingers. Your body temperature will slowly dissolve the suppository and release the medicine across your rectum and into the bloodstream.
- Empty your bowels if necessary.
- Wash and dry your hands.
- Remove the suppository from its foil or wrapper.
- Lie down on your side with one leg bent and the other straight.
- Carefully push the suppository 2–3 cm up your bottom, pointed end first, using your finger. Some people may prefer to wear a glove, but this is not necessary.
- Close your legs and lie still for a few minutes.
- Wash your hands afterwards.
- If you open your bowels within 2 hours after inserting the suppository, you need to insert another.
- The suppository may leak from your rectum, so it may be best to insert it before bedtime and (if female) to use a sanitary towel to avoid staining of the clothes.
- If you miss a dose, insert the suppository as soon as you remember, and then carry on as normal.
- Check the expiry date before using your suppository.
- Store in a cool, dark place and out of children's reach.
- Continue using your suppositories until the course is completed.

After the explanation

- Summarise and check the patient's understanding.
- Ask if she/he has any questions or concerns.
- Offer her/him a leaflet.

Station 77

Rheumatological history

Before starting

- Introduce yourself to the patient.
- Explain that you are going to ask him some questions to uncover the nature of his complaint, and ask him for his consent to do this.
- Ensure that he is comfortable.

The history

Name, age, and occupation, if this information has not already been supplied.

Presenting complaint

Ask the patient about the nature of his complaint.

Pain

Ask specifically about any pain and determine its site (i.e. which joints are affected), characteristics, and timing. Is there any swelling?

Stiffness

Ask specifically about difficulty in starting or carrying out movement.

History of presenting complaint

Ask about:

- The circumstances of disease onset.
- The subsequent course of the disease.
- Any associated features:
  - local: inflammation, deformity, cracking, clicking, locking, loss of movement
  - systemic: skin problems, eye problems, GI disturbances
  - general: malaise, fever, weight loss
- Possible trauma or infection.

Social history

- Ask the patient whether he is finding it difficult to complete everyday tasks and, if so, what effect this is having on his life. You might get him to describe a typical day: getting out of bed, toileting, dressing, etc. What things could he do before that he can now no longer do?
- Ask about housing and home-help.
- Ask about mood, and about some of the key features of depression such as low mood, fatigu-ability and loss of interest.
- Also ask about travel.

Past medical history

- Current, past, and childhood illnesses.

- Surgery.
- Recent visits to the doctor.

Drug history

- Prescribed medication, e.g. NSAIDs, steroids, immunosuppressants.
- Over-the-counter medications.
- Allergies.
- Smoking, alcohol use, and recreational drug use.

Family history

- Parents, siblings, children. Has anyone in the family ever had similar problems?

After taking the history

- Ask the patient if there is anything he might add that you have forgotten to ask about.
- Thank the patient.

Most common conditions likely to come up in a rheumatological history station	
Rheumatoid arthritis	Septic arthritis
Osteoarthritis	Polymyositis or dermatomyositis
Psoriatic arthritis	Polymyalgia rheumatica
Gout or pseudo-gout	Tendon rupture
Ankylosing spondylitis	Complications of steroid treatment

Station 78

The GALS screening examination

GALS: 'Gait, arms, legs, and spine'. Remember that GALS is a screening test and that a detailed examination should therefore not be required.

Before starting

- Introduce yourself to the patient.
- Explain the examination and ask for his consent to carry it out.
- Ask him to undress to his undergarments.
- Ensure that he is comfortable.

The GALS screening examination

Brief history

- Name, age, and occupation, if this information has not already been supplied.
- *"Do you have any pain or stiffness in your muscles, back, or joints?"*
- *"Do you have any difficulty in climbing stairs?"*
- *"Do you have any difficulty washing or dressing?"*

The examination

General inspection

Inspect the patient standing. Note any obvious scars, swellings, deformities, and/or unusual posturing.

Spine

Look

- From the front.
- From behind, looking in particular for lumbar lordosis and scoliosis.
- From the side, looking in particular for kyphosis and fixed flexion deformity.

Feel

- Press on each vertebral body in turn, trying to elicit tenderness.

Move

- Ask the patient to bend forwards and touch his toes. Look for loss of lumbar lordosis, scoliosis (it usually becomes more pronounced), and the normal range of movement.

Ask the patient to sit down on the couch.

- Lateral flexion of the neck. *"Put your ear on your shoulder."*
- Flexion and extension of the neck. *"Put your chin on your chest."*
- Spinal rotation. *"Turn your upper body to either side."*

Demonstrate each of these movements to the patient. In particular, look for restricted range of movement and pain on movement.

Arms

Look

- Skin: rashes, nodules, nail signs
- Muscles: wasting, fasciculation
- Joints: swelling, asymmetry, deformity

 Do not forget to inspect both surfaces of the hands.

Feel

- Skin: temperature
- Muscles: general muscle bulk
- Joints: tenderness and warmth; squeeze each hand at the level of the carpal and meta-carpal joints, and try to localise any tenderness by squeezing each individual joint in turn

Move

- Hands: 1. power grip: test the strength of the grip by asking the patient to squeeze your finger
                2. precision pinch grip: test the strength of the grip by trying to 'break' the patient's pinch
- Wrists: flexion and extension
- Elbows: flexion and extension
- Shoulders: full external rotation and abduction (hands behind the head)

Demonstrate these movements to the patient. Note if there is a restricted range of movement and/or any pain on movement.

Legs

Now ask the patient to lie on the couch.

Look

- Skin: rashes, nodules, callosities on the soles of the feet
- Muscles: wasting, fasciculation
- Joints: swelling, asymmetry, deformity

Feel

- Skin: temperature
- Joints: tenderness, warmth, and swelling; palpate each knee along the joint margin; squeeze each foot, and try to localise any tenderness by squeezing each individual joint in turn

Move

- Bend each knee in turn.
- Hold the knee and hip at 90 degrees of flexion and internally and externally rotate the hip. Keep an eye on the patient's face as you do this and ensure that you do not cause the patient unnecessary pain.
- Next, place one hand on the knee joint and extend it, feeling for any crepitus as you do so.

Gait

Ask the patient to walk, observing:

- general features: rhythm, speed, limp, turning
- the phases of gait: heel-strike, stance, push-off, and swing
- transfer ability: sitting and standing from a chair (note that you should already have had a chance to observe this)

After the examination

- Thank the patient.
- Offer to help the patient dress.
- Ensure that he is comfortable.
- Summarise your findings.

Hand and wrist examination

Before starting

- Introduce yourself to the patient.
- Explain the examination and ask for his consent to carry it out.
- Ask him to expose his arms.
- Ensure that he is comfortable.

The examination

Look

First inspect the dorsum and then the palmar surfaces of the hands.

- Skin: colour, rheumatoid nodules, scars, nail changes.
- Joints: swelling, Heberden's nodes, Bouchard's nodes.
- Shape and position: normal resting position of the hand, ulnar deviation, boutonnière and swan neck deformity of the fingers, mallet finger, finger droop, Z-deformity of the thumb, muscle wasting, Dupuytren's contracture.

Boutonnière deformity

Swan neck deformity

Figure 52. The arthritic hand. Boutonnière and swan neck deformity of the fingers.

Feel

Ask if the hands are painful.

- Skin: temperature.
- Finger and wrist joints: swelling, synovial thickening, tenderness.
- Anatomical snuff box (fractured scaphoid).
- Tip of the radial styloid and head of the ulna.

Move

Test active and passive movements, looking for limitation in the normal range of movement. Ask the patient to report any pain.

Wrist

- Flexion and extension.
- Ulnar and radial deviation.
- Pronation and supination.

Thumb

- Extension. *"Stick your thumb out to the side."*
- Abduction. *"Point your thumb up to the ceiling."*
- Adduction. *"Collect your thumb in your palm."*
- Opposition. *"Appose the tip of your thumb to the tip of your little finger."*

Fingers

Each finger should be fully extended and flexed. Look at the movements of the metacarpophalangeal and interphalangeal joints. Test the grip strength by asking the patient to make a fist and try to squeeze your fingers. Try to open the fist. Test the pincer strength by trying to break the pinch between his thumb and first finger.

Special tests

- Carpal tunnel tests:
  - try to elicit Tinnel's sign by extending the hand and tapping on the median nerve in the carpal tunnel
  - try to elicit Phalen's sign by holding the hand in forced flexion for 30–60 seconds

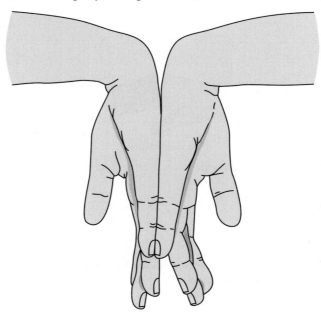

Figure 53. An alternative and quicker method for eliciting Phalen's sign.

- *Flexor profundus*: hold a finger extended at the proximal interphalangeal joint and ask the patient to flex the distal interphalangeal joint of that same finger.

- *Flexor superficialis*: ask the patient to flex a finger whilst holding all the other fingers on the same hand extended.
- Assess function by asking the patient to make use of an everyday object such as a pen or cup.

After the examination

- State that you would also like to examine the vascular and neurological systems of the upper limb.
- If appropriate, indicate that you would order some tests, e.g. X-ray, FBC, ESR, rheumatoid factor, etc.
- Thank the patient.
- Ensure that he is comfortable.
- Offer to help the patient put his clothes back on.
- Offer a differential diagnosis.

Most common conditions likely to come up in a hand and wrist examination station	
Osteoarthritis	Gout
Rheumatoid arthritis	Dupuytren's disease
Psoriatic arthritis – look at the nails!	De Quervain's tenosynovitis
Lesions of the median, radial, or ulnar nerves	Trigger finger

Figure 54. Rheumatoid arthritis of the hands.

Reproduced from www.mrcophth.com.

Station 80

Elbow examination

This station is unlikely to come up on its own but may be asked as part of a hand and wrist examination, and is included here for completeness.

Before starting

- Introduce yourself to the patient.
- Explain the examination and ask for his consent to carry it out.
- Ask him to expose his arms.
- Ensure that he is comfortable.

The examination

Look

Ask the patient to hold his arms by his side.

- Overall impression: varus or valgus deformities (look from behind), effusions, inflammation of the olecranon bursa
- Skin: rheumatoid nodules, gouty tophi, scars
- Muscle wasting: biceps, triceps, forearm

Feel

Ask if the arms are painful.

- Skin: temperature, rheumatoid nodules, gouty tophi
- Joints: tenderness, effusions, synovial thickening
- Bones: tenderness of the lateral and medial epicondyles

Move

- Flexion and extension:
  - tennis elbow: ask about pain at the *lateral* epicondyle on elbow *extension* and forced wrist *extension*
  - golfer's elbow: ask about pain at the *medial* epicondyle on elbow *flexion* and forced wrist *flexion*
- Pronation and supination. Show the patient how to tuck his elbows into his sides and to turn his arms so that the palm of his hands face up and down (a bit like the gesture for 'I don't know').

After the examination

- State that you would also like to examine the wrist and hand.
- State that you would also like to examine the vascular and neurological systems of the upper limb.
- If appropriate, indicate that you would order some tests, e.g. X-ray, FBC, ESR, rheumatoid factor, etc.
- Thank the patient.
- Offer to help the patient put his clothes back on.
- Ensure that he is comfortable.
- Summarise your findings and offer a differential diagnosis.

Most common conditions likely to come up in an elbow examination station

Osteoarthritis

Rheumatoid arthritis

Olecranon bursitis

Station 81

Shoulder examination

Before starting

- Introduce yourself to the patient.
- Explain the examination and ask for his consent to carry it out.
- Ask him to undress from the waist upward.
- Ensure that he is comfortable.

The examination

Look

Inspect from front and back.

- Overall impression: alignment, position of the arms, axillae, prominence of the acromio-clavicular and sternoclavicular joints
- Skin: colour, sinuses, scars
- Muscle wasting: deltoid, periscapular muscles (supraspinatus and infraspinatus)

Feel

Ask if the shoulders are painful.

- Skin: temperature
- Bones and joints: palpate the bony landmarks of the shoulder, starting at the sternoclavicular joint and moving laterally along the clavicle. Try to localise any tenderness. Can you feel any effusions?
- Biceps tendon.

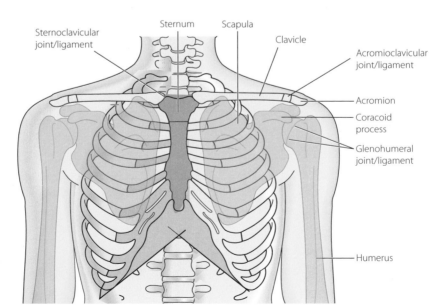

Figure 55. Anatomy of the shoulder joint.

Orthopaedics and rheumatology

Move

Demonstrate these movements to the patient. Note if there is a restricted range of movement and/ or any pain on movement.

- Abduction:
  Raise your arms above your head, making the palms of your hands touch.
- Adduction:
  Cross your arms across the front of your body.
- Flexion:
  Raise your arms forwards.
- Extension:
  Pull your arms backwards.
- External rotation:
  With your arms bent and your elbows tucked into your sides separate your hands.
- Internal rotation:
  With your arms bent and your elbows tucked into your sides bring your hands together.
- Internal rotation in adduction:
  Reach up your back and touch your scapulae.
- External rotation in abduction:
  Hold your hands behind your neck, like you do at the end of the day.

 If any one movement is limited, also test the passive range of movement.

Serratus anterior function

Ask the patient to put his hands against a wall and to push against it. Observe the scapulae from behind, looking for asymmetry or winging.

After the examination

- State that you would also like to examine the vascular and neurological systems of the upper limb.
- If appropriate, indicate that you would order some tests, e.g. X-ray, FBC, ESR, rheumatoid factor, etc.
- Thank the patient.
- Offer to help the patient put his clothes back on.
- Ensure that he is comfortable.
- Summarise your findings and offer a differential diagnosis.

Most common conditions likely to come up in a shoulder examination OSCE
Frozen shoulder
Acute calcific tendonitis
Rotator cuff tear
Winging of the scapula
Bicipital tendonitis
Osteoarthritis
Referred pain from the cervical spine or the heart
Rupture of the long head of biceps (look out for Popeye's sign!)

Station 82

Spinal examination

Before starting

- Introduce yourself to the patient.
- Explain the examination and ask for his consent to carry it out.
- Ask him to undress to his undergarments.
- Ensure that he is comfortable.

The examination

Look

Inspect from front and back.

- General inspection: ask the patient to stand and assess posture. Are there any obvious mal-formations?
- Skin: scars, pigmentation, abnormal hair, unusual skin creases.
- Shape and posture.
- Spine:
  - lateral curvature of the spine – *scoliosis* (observe from the back)
  - abnormal increase in the kyphotic curvature of the thoracic spine – *kyphosis* (observe from the side)
  - sharp, angular bend in the spine – a *kyphos* (observe from the side)
  - loss or exaggeration of lumbar lordosis
- Asymmetry or malformation of the chest.
- Asymmetry of the pelvis.

Feel

Ask if there is any pain.

- Palpate and percuss the spinous processes, the interspinous ligaments, and the paravertebral muscles.

Move

Ask the patient to copy your movements, looking for any limitation of range of movement. Ask the patient to indicate if any of the movements are painful.

Gait

Cervical spine

- Flexion.
- Extension.
- Lateral flexion.
- Rotation (look back over each shoulder).

Thoracic spine

- Rotation (twist from side to side – ask the patient to sit or stabilise his pelvis).

Measure chest expansion. It should be at least 5 cm.

Lumbar spine

- Flexion. *Touch your toes, keep your knees straight.*
- Extension. *Lean back, keep your knees straight.*
- Lateral flexion. *Slide your hand alongside the outside of your leg.*

Measure lumbar excursion by drawing a line from 10 cm above L5 to 5 cm below it and asking the patient to bend fully forwards. Extension of the line by <5 cm indicates movement restriction.

Special tests

Ask the patient to lie prone.

- Palpate the sacroiliac joints for tenderness.
- Press on the mid-line of the sacrum to test if movement of the sacroiliac joints is painful.
- Femoral stretch test (L2–L4):
  - flex the knee
  - if this does not trigger any pain, extend the leg at the hip – pain suggests irritation of the second, third, or fourth lumbar root of that side

Figure 56. The femoral stretch test.

Ask the patient to lie supine.

- Straight leg raise (sciatica, L5–S2):
  - flex the hip while maintaining the knee in extension
  - pain in the thigh, buttock, and back suggests sciatica
  - the response can be amplified by concomitant dorsiflexion of the foot (Bragard's test)
  - perform Lasegue's test if you're after a gold medal! With the hip and knee flexed to 90 degrees, and your left hand on the knee, extend the knee with your right hand.

After the examination

- State that you would also like to carry out neurological and vascular examinations.
- If appropriate, indicate that you would order some tests, e.g. X-ray, MRI, DEXA, FBC, ESR, bone profile, etc.
- Thank the patient.
- Offer to help the patient put his clothes back on.
- Ensure that he is comfortable.
- Summarise your findings and offer a differential diagnosis.

Most common conditions likely to come up in a spinal examination station

Ankylosing spondylitis	Scoliosis
Muscular back pain	Prolapsed disc
Osteoarthritis	

Hip examination

Before starting

- Introduce yourself to the patient.
- Explain the examination and ask for his consent to carry it out.
- Ask him to undress to his undergarments.
- Ensure that he is comfortable.

The examination

Look

Inspect from front and back.

- General inspection: posture, symmetry of legs and pelvis, deformity, muscle wasting, scars.
- Gait (observe from the front and back). Note any limp – antalgic, short leg, or Trendelenberg.
- Trendelenberg's test: ask the patient to stand on each leg in turn, lifting the other one off the ground by bending it at the knee. Face the patient and support him by the index fingers of his outstretched hands. The sign is positive if the pelvis drops on the unsupported side.

Figure 57. Negative (left) and positive Trendelenberg's test. A positive Trendelenberg's test suggests that the weight-bearing hip is either painful or has a weak gluteus medius.

Ask the patient to lie supine.

- Skin: colour, sinuses, scars.
- Position: limb shortening, limb rotation, abduction or adduction deformity, flexion deformity.
- Limb length.
  - To measure *true* leg length, position the pelvis so that the iliac crests lie in the same horizontal plane, at right angles to the trunk (this is not possible if there is a fixed abduction or adduction deformity) and then measure the distance from the anterior superior iliac spine (ASIS) to the medial malleolus. True leg shortening suggests pathology of the hip joint.
  - To measure *apparent* leg length, measure the distance from the xiphisternum to the medial malleolus. Apparent leg shortening suggests pelvic tilt, most often due to an adduction deformity of the hip.
- Circumference of the quadriceps muscles at a fixed point.

Feel

Ask if there is any pain.

- Skin: temperature, effusions (difficult to feel).
- Bones and joints: bony landmarks of the hip joint, inguinal ligament.

Move

Look for limitation of the normal range of movement, and ask the patient to report any pain.

- Flexion and Thomas' test:
  - flex both hips and place your hand in the small of the back to ensure that the lumbar lordosis has been eliminated
  - hold one hip flexed and straighten the other leg, maintaining your hand in the small of the back – if the leg cannot be straightened and the knee is unable to rest on the couch, a fixed flexion deformity is present
  - repeat for the other leg
- Abduction and adduction:
  - drop one leg over the edge of the couch to fix the pelvis
  - place one hand on the anterior superior iliac spine of the other leg and carry it through abduction and adduction
  - repeat for the other leg
- Rotation:
  - flex the hip and knee to 90 degrees
  - hold the knee in the left hand and the ankle in the right hand
  - using your right hand, rotate the hip internally and externally
  - repeat for the other leg

Ask the patient to lie prone.

- Look for scars, etc.
- Feel for tenderness.
- Extend each hip in turn. Keep a hand under a bent knee and extend the hip by pulling the leg up at the ankle.

After the examination

- State that you would also like to examine the vascular and neurological systems of the lower limbs.

- If appropriate, indicate that you would order some tests, e.g. hip and knee X-ray, DEXA, FBC, ESR, bone profile, etc.
- Thank the patient.
- Offer to help the patient put his clothes back on.
- Ensure that he is comfortable.
- Summarise your findings and offer a differential diagnosis.

Most common conditions likely to come up in a hip examination station
Osteoarthritis: hip in flexion, external rotation, and adduction, apparent limb shortening, pain, limp, limited range of movement, Heberden's nodes on distal interphalangeal joints
Hip replacement
Hip arthrodesis
Slipped upper femoral epiphysis
Trendelenburg gait
Antalgic gait

Knee examination

Before starting

- Introduce yourself to the patient.
- Explain the examination and ask for his consent to carry it out.
- Ask him to undress from the waist downwards.
- Ensure that he is comfortable.

The examination

Ask the patient to stand.

Look

- Gait: observe from in front and behind, looking for instability, limp, and limited range of movement.
- Position: neutral, varus, valgus, fixed flexion, hyperextension (recurvatum).
- Squat test (avoid in elderly patients).

Ask the patient to lie supine.

- Skin: colour, sinuses, scars (including arthroscopic scars).
- Shape: alignment, effusion, patellar alignment.
- Position: hyperextension, varus, valgus.

Measure quadriceps circumference a hand breadth above the patella.

Feel

Ask if there is any pain.

- Skin: temperature (compare both sides).
- Effusions: patellar tap test, cross fluctuation, and bulge test.
- Joint line at 90 degrees of flexion.
- Synovial thickening.
- Surrounding structures: ligaments, tibial tuberosity, femoral condyles.
- Patella: note size and height and carry out patellar friction and patellar apprehension tests (displace the patella laterally as you flex the knee).

Move

- Active:
  - flexion
  - extension
- Passive:
  - flexion (to 140 degrees), feeling for crepitus and clicks
  - extension (to 0 to −10 degrees)
- Straight leg raise.

Special tests

- Collateral ligament tears.
  - Apply varus and valgus stresses at 0 degrees and 20 degrees of flexion. Hold the leg under one arm and apply pressure on the medial/lateral side of the knee joint.
- Cruciate ligament tears.
  - Posterior sag test: flex the knee to 90 degrees and look for a sag across the knee. The presence of a sag indicates a posterior cruciate ligament tear.
  - Anterior and posterior drawer tests: flex the knee to 90 degrees, sit on the foot (ask the patient first!), and pull the tibia back and forth.
  - Lachman's test: flex the knee to 30 degrees and, holding the thigh in one hand and the proximal tibia in the other, attempt to make the joint surfaces slide on one another.

Figure 58. Lachman's test.

- Meniscal tears.
  - McMurray's test: place one hand on the knee and the other on the ankle. Flex the hip and knee. To test the medial meniscus, palpate the posteromedial margin of the joint. Then hold the leg in external rotation and extend the knee. To test the lateral meniscus, palpate the posterolateral margin of the joint. Then hold the leg in internal rotation and extend the knee. A positive test is one that elicits pain, resistance, or a reproducible click.
  - Apley's grinding test (not usually performed).

Figure 59. McMurray's test.

Lie the patient prone.

- Popliteal fossa:
  - inspect the popliteal fossa
  - palpate the popliteal fossa for a Baker's (popliteal) cyst

After the examination

- State that you would also like to examine the vascular and neurological systems of the lower limbs.
- If appropriate, indicate that you would order some tests, e.g. knee X-ray, FBC, ESR, bone profile, rheumatoid factor, etc.
- Thank the patient.
- Offer to help the patient put his clothes back on.
- Ensure that he is comfortable.
- Summarise your findings and offer a differential diagnosis.

 The age and sex of the patient have a strong bearing on the differential diagnosis.

Most common conditions likely to come up in a knee examination station	
Osteoarthritis	Recurrent subluxation of the patella
Rheumatoid arthritis	Tibial apophysitis (Osgood–Schlätter's disease)
Baker's (popliteal) cyst	Collateral ligament tears
Prepatellar and infrapatellar bursitis	Cruciate ligament tears
Chrondromalacia patellae	Meniscal tears

Ankle and foot examination

Before starting

- Introduce yourself to the patient.
- Explain the examination and ask for his consent to carry it out.
- Ask him to undress from the waist downwards.
- Ensure that he is comfortable.

The examination

The patient is standing.

Look

- General inspection: posture, symmetry, and any obvious deformities. Ask the patient to turn around.
- Gait: observe from front and back. Ask the patient to stand on his tiptoes and then on his heels.

Ask the patient to lie on the couch.

- Skin: colour, sinuses, scars, corns, calluses, ulcers.
- Shape: alignment, *pes planus* (flat foot), *pes cavus* (arched foot), deformities of the toes (*hallux valgus*, claw, hammer, and mallet toes).
- Position: varus or valgus hindfoot deformity.

Figure 60. Claw, mallet, and hammer toes.

Feel

Ask about any pain.

- Skin: temperature (compare both sides), abnormal thickening on the soles of the feet.
- Pulses: dorsalis pedis, posterior tibial.
- Bone and joints: palpate the joint margin, forefoot (metatarsals and metatarsophalangeal joints) and hindfoot, and localise any tenderness. Remember to keep looking at the patient's face.

Move

Look for restriction of the normal range of movement. Ask the patient to report any pain.

Ankle joint

- Hold the heel in the left hand and the forefoot in the right hand.
- Plantarflex the foot (normal range 40 degrees).
- Dorsiflex the foot (normal range 25 degrees).
- Compare range of movement to that in the other foot.

Subtalar joint

- Hold the heel in the left hand and the forefoot in the right hand, as above, with the ankle fixed at 90 degrees.
- Invert the foot (normal range 30 degrees).
- Evert the foot (normal range 30 degrees).
- Compare the range of movement to that in the other foot.

Midtarsal joint

- Hold the heel in the left hand and the forefoot in the right hand.
- Flex, extend, invert, and evert the forefoot.

Toes

- Flex and extend each toe in turn. If there is any tenderness, try to localise it to a particular joint.

Ask the patient to lie prone.

- Look for any scars and for wasting of the calves.
- Palpate the calf muscle and the Achilles' tendon (*tendo calcaneus*).
- Simmond's test: squeeze the calf – if the foot plantarflexes, the tendo calcaneus is intact.

After the examination

- State that you would also like to examine the vascular and neurological systems of the lower limbs.
- If appropriate, indicate that you would order some tests, e.g. foot and ankle X-ray, FBC, ESR, bone profile, rheumatoid factor, etc.
- Thank the patient.
- Offer to help the patient put his socks and shoes back on.
- Ensure that he is comfortable.
- Summarise your findings and offer a differential diagnosis.

Most common conditions likely to come up in an ankle and foot examination station	
Osteoarthritis	Deformities of the foot
Rheumatoid arthritis	Plantar fasciitis
Ankle injuries	

Orthopaedics and rheumatology

Figure 61. Hallux (abducto) valgus.

Reproduced from http://commons.wikimedia.org – photograph by Dr Henri Lelièvre.

Station 86

Adult Basic Life Support

- Make sure the victim, any bystanders, and you are safe.
- Check the victim for a response. Gently shake his shoulders and ask loudly, *Are you all right?*

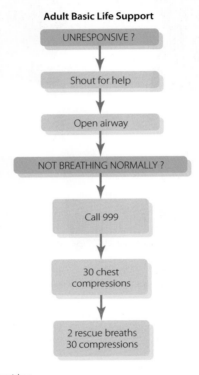

Adult Basic Life Support

UNRESPONSIVE ?

↓

Shout for help

↓

Open airway

↓

NOT BREATHING NORMALLY ?

↓

Call 999

↓

30 chest compressions

↓

2 rescue breaths
30 compressions

Figure 62. Basic Life Support algorithm.

If he responds:

- Leave him in the position in which you find him provided there is no further danger.
- Try to find out what is wrong with him and get help if needed.
- Reassess him regularly.

If he does not respond:

- Shout for help.
- Turn him onto his back and open the airway using the head-tilt, chin-lift technique.
  - Place your hand on his forehead and gently tilt his head back.
  - With your fingertips under the point of his chin, lift the chin to open the airway.
  - Holding his airway open, put your ear to his mouth. *Listen, feel,* and *look* for breathing for no more than 10 seconds. If you have any doubt about whether breathing is normal, assume that it is not.

 Agonal breathing (occasional gasps, slow, laboured, or noisy breathing) is common in the early stages of cardiac arrest and should not be mistaken for a sign of life.

Figure 63. The head-tilt, chin-lift technique.

If he is breathing normally:

- Turn him into the recovery position.
- Send or go for help, or call for an ambulance.
- Check for continued breathing.

If he is not breathing normally:

- Ask someone to call for an ambulance or, if you are on your own, do this yourself: you may need to leave the victim.
- Deliver 30 chest compressions followed by 2 rescue breaths.
  To deliver chest compressions:
  - kneel by the side of the victim
  - place the heel of one hand in the centre of the victim's chest
  - place the heel of the other hand on top of the first hand
  - interlock the fingers of your hands and ensure that pressure is not applied on the victim's ribs, bottom end of his chest bone, or upper abdomen
  - position yourself vertically above the victim's chest and, with your arms straight, press down on the sternum 4–5 cm
  - after each compression, release all the pressure on the chest without losing contact between your hands and the sternum – repeat at a rate of about 100 per minute
  - compression and release should take an equal amount of time
  To deliver rescue breaths:
  - after 30 compressions, again open the airway using head tilt and chin lift
  - pinch the soft part of the victim's nose closed using the index finger and thumb of the hand on his forehead
  - allow his mouth to open, but maintain chin lift
  - take a normal breath and place your lips around his mouth, making sure that you have a good seal
  - blow steadily into his mouth whilst watching for his chest to rise – take about 1 second to make his chest rise
  - maintaining head tilt and chin lift, take your mouth away from him and watch for his chest to fall
  - deliver a second rescue breath and return to chest compressions without delay
- Continue with chest compressions and rescue breaths at a ratio of 30:2.
- Stop to re-check the victim only if he starts breathing normally.
- If your rescue breaths do not make the chest rise as in normal breathing, check the victim's mouth and remove any obstruction and re-check that there is adequate head tilt and

chin lift. Do not attempt more than 2 rescue breaths each time before returning to chest compressions.

- If there is more than one rescuer present, another should take over CPR every 2 minutes to prevent fatigue.

 If the rescuer is unable or unwilling to give rescue breaths, he can give chest compressions at a rate of 100 compressions per minute, stopping only to recheck the victim if he starts breathing normally.

Continue resuscitation until qualified help arrives or until the victim starts breathing normally or until exhaustion.

The recovery position

- Remove the victim's spectacles, if any.
- Kneel beside the victim and make sure that both his legs are straight.
- Place the arm nearest to you out at right angles to his body, elbow bent, with the hand palm uppermost.
- Bring the far arm across the chest, and hold the back of the hand against the victim's cheek nearest to you.
- With your other hand, grasp the far leg just above the knee and pull it up, keeping the foot on the ground.
- Keeping his hand pressed against his cheek, pull on the far leg to roll the victim towards you and onto his side.
- Adjust the upper leg so that both the hip and knee are bent at right angles.
- Tilt the head back to ensure that the airway remains open.
- Adjust the hand under the cheek, if necessary, to keep the head tilted.

Figure 64. The recovery position.

Emergency medicine and anaesthesiology

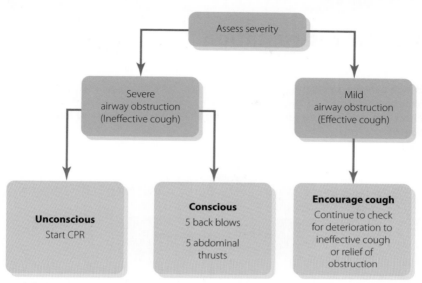

Figure 65. Adult choking algorithm.

Adapted from Resuscitation Council (UK) 2005 Guidelines.

In-hospital resuscitation

This sequence should be followed for a collapsed patient in hospital.

- Ensure personal safety.
- Shout for help.
- Check the patient for a response – gently shake his shoulders and loudly ask *Are you all right?*

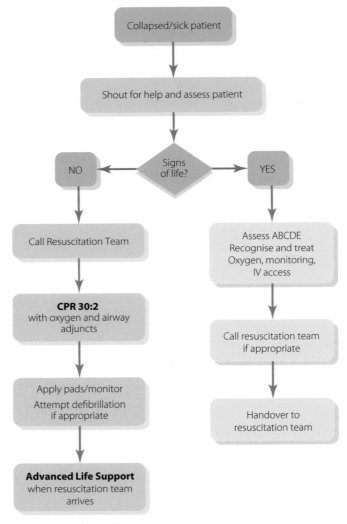

Figure 66. In-hospital resuscitation algorithm.

- If the patient responds:
  - urgent medical assessment is required – depending on local protocols, this may be by the resuscitation team

- while awaiting the arrival of this team, assess the patient using the ABCDE approach
- give the patient oxygen
- attach monitoring leads
- obtain venous access
- If the patient does not respond:
  - turn the patient onto his back
  - open the airway using the head-tilt, chin-lift technique
  - look into the mouth – if a foreign body or debris is visible, attempt to remove it using suction or forceps as appropriate
  - if there is a risk of C-spine injury, use the jaw-thrust or chin-lift technique with manual in-line stabilisation (MILS) of the head and neck by an assistant (if sufficient staff are available). If airway obstruction persists despite jaw thrust or chin lift, add head tilt a small amount at a time. Establishing an airway should take priority over concerns about a potential C-spine injury.
- Holding the patient's airway open, put your ear to his mouth. *Listen, feel,* and *look* for breathing for no more than 10 seconds.
- Assess the carotid pulse at the same time or after the breathing check.

Figure 67. The head-tilt jaw-thrust technique.

 Agonal breathing (occasional gasps, slow, laboured, or noisy breathing) is common in the early stages of cardiac arrest and should not be mistaken for a sign of life.

- If the patient has a pulse or other signs of life.
  - Urgent medical assessment is required. Depending on local protocols, this may be by the resuscitation team.
  - While awaiting the arrival of this team, assess the patient using the ABCDE approach.
  - Give the patient oxygen.
  - Attach monitoring leads.
  - Obtain venous access.
- If there is no pulse or other signs of life.
  - One person should start CPR as others call the resuscitation team or collect the resuscitation equipment. If only one member of staff is present, this will mean leaving the patient.
  - Give 30 chest compressions followed by 2 ventilations. Place your interlocked hands in the middle of the lower half of the sternum and depress the chest by 4–5 cm, aiming for a rate of 100 compressions per minute.
  - Maintain the airway and ventilate the lungs with the most appropriate equipment immediately at hand. A pocket mask, which may be supplemented by an oral airway, is usually

    readily available. If no equipment is immediately at hand, give mouth-to-mouth ventilation unless there are clinical reasons to avoid mouth-to-mouth contact.

- Use an inspiratory time of 1 second and give enough volume to produce a chest rise as in normal breathing. Add supplemental oxygen as soon as possible.
- Once the airway has been secured, continue chest compressions uninterrupted at a rate of 100 compressions per minute and ventilate the lungs at approximately 10 breaths per minute. Only stop compressions for defibrillation or pulse checks.
- Upon arrival of the defibrillator, apply the paddles to the patient and analyse the rhythm. The use of adhesive electrode pads or the 'quick look' paddles technique enables rapid assessment of the heart rhythm compared to attaching ECG electrodes.
- If self-adhesive defibrillation pads are available and there is more than one rescuer, apply the pads without interrupting chest compression. Pause briefly to assess rhythm and, if indicated, proceed to either manual or automated defibrillation.
- Recommence chest compressions immediately after the first attempt at defibrillation. Do not pause to assess the pulse or heart rhythm.
- Continue resuscitation until the resuscitation team arrives or until the patient shows signs of life. If using an automated external defibrillator (AED), follow the voice prompts. If using a manual defibrillator, follow the algorithm for ALS (see next station).
- Once resuscitation is underway, and if there are sufficient people available, prepare intravenous cannulae and drugs that are likely to be needed by the resuscitation team.
- Identify one person to be responsible for handover to the resuscitation team leader. Locate the patient's notes.
- Change the person providing chest compressions every 2 minutes to prevent fatigue.

- If the patient is not breathing but has a pulse (respiratory arrest).
  - Ventilate the patient's lungs as described above, checking for a pulse after every 10 breaths (about every minute).
  - If there are any doubts about the presence of a pulse, start chest compressions until more experienced help arrives.
- If a patient has a monitored and witnessed cardiac arrest.
  - Confirm cardiac arrest and shout for help.
  - After confirmation of VF/VT cardiac arrest, deliver a first shock.
  - If a defibrillator is not immediately to hand, consider giving a single precordial thump immediately after confirmation of VF/VT cardiac arrest.
  - Start CPR (as described above) immediately after the first shock is delivered.
  - Continue resuscitation in accordance with the algorithm for ALS.

Adapted from Resuscitation Council (UK) 2005 Guidelines.

Advanced Life Support

Specifications: A mannequin in lieu of a patient.

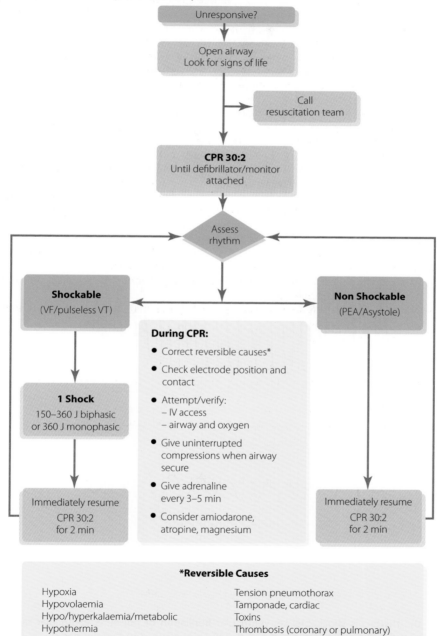

Figure 68. Advanced Life Support algorithm.

The patient has arrested and CPR is under way. The defibrillator/monitor has just been attached.

Figure 69. Positioning of the defibrillator paddles.

- **Assess the rhythm.**

Ventricular tachycardia

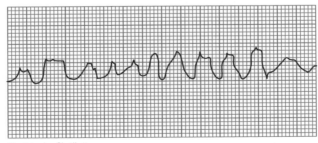

Ventricular fibrillation

Figure 70. ECG traces of ventricular fibrillation and ventricular tachycardia.

- If the rhythm is shockable, i.e. ventricular fibrillation or pulseless ventricular tachycardia, attempt defibrillation (one shock – 150–200 J biphasic or 360 J monophasic).

Remember to shout "All clear" and "Oxygen away", and to perform a visual check of the area each time you attempt defibrillation.

- Immediately resume CPR with chest compressions (30:2) without reassessing the rhythm or feeling for a pulse.
- Continue CPR for 2 minutes then pause briefly to check the monitor.
- If VF/VT persists:
  - immediately deliver a second shock (150–360 J biphasic or 360 J monophasic)
  - resume CPR immediately and continue for 2 minutes
  - pause briefly to check the monitor
- If VF/VT still persists:
  - give adrenaline 1 mg IV
  - immediately deliver a third shock (150–360 J biphasic or 360 J monophasic)
  - resume CPR immediately and continue for 2 minutes
  - pause briefly to check the monitor
- If VF/VT still persists:
  - give amiodarone 300 mg IV
  - immediately deliver a fourth shock (150–360 J biphasic or 360 J monophasic)
  - resume CPR immediately and continue for 2 minutes
  - give adrenaline 1 mg IV immediately before alternate shocks (i.e. approximately every 3–5 minutes)
  - deliver a further shock after each 2 minute period of CPR and after confirming that VF/VT persists
  - if organised electrical activity is seen during this brief pause in compressions, check for a pulse
  - if a pulse is present, start post-resuscitation care
  - if a pulse is absent, continue CPR and switch to the non-shockable algorithm

During CPR, seek to
• Correct reversible causes*.
• Check electrode position and contact.
• Attempt/verify: IV access, airway, and oxygen.
• Give uninterrupted compressions when the airway is secure.
• Give adrenaline every 3–5 minutes.
• Consider: amiodarone, atropine, magnesium.

*Reversible causes:

Hypoxia	**T**ension pneumothorax
Hypovolaemia	**T**amponade
Hypo/hyperkalaemia, metabolic	**T**oxins
Hypothermia	**T**hrombosis (coronary or pulmonary)

Precordial thump

If a patient has a monitored and witnessed cardiac arrest and a defibrillator is not immediately to hand, consider giving a single precordial thump immediately after confirmation of VF/VT cardiac arrest. Using the ulnar edge of a tightly clenched fist, deliver a sharp impact to the lower half of the sternum from a height of about 20 cm, then retract the fist immediately to create an impulse-like stimulus. A precordial thump is most likely to be successful in converting VT to sinus rhythm.

Non-shockable rhythms (PEA and asystole)

Survival after cardiac arrest with PEA or asystole is unlikely unless a reversible cause can be found and treated successfully.

Sequence of actions for PEA (cardiac electrical activity in the absence of any palpable pulse).

- Start CPR 30:2.
- Give adrenaline 1 mg IV as soon as IV access is achieved.
- Continue CPR 30:2 until the airway is secured, then continue chest compressions without pausing during ventilation.
- Recheck the rhythm after 2 minutes.
- If there is no change in the ECG appearance:
  - continue CPR
  - recheck the rhythm after 2 minutes and proceed accordingly
  - give further adrenaline 1 mg IV after every 3–5 minutes (alternate loops)
- If the ECG changes and organized electrical activity is seen, check for a pulse.
- If a pulse is present, start post-resuscitation care.
- If no pulse is present:
  - continue CPR
  - recheck the rhythm after 2 minutes and proceed accordingly
  - give further adrenaline 1 mg IV after every 3–5 minutes (alternate loops)

Sequence of actions for asystole and slow PEA (rate < 60 per minute).

- Start CPR 30:2.
- Without stopping CPR, check that the leads are attached correctly.
- Give adrenaline 1 mg IV as soon as IV access is achieved.
- Give atropine 3 mg IV (once only).
- Continue CPR 30:2 until the airway is secured, then continue chest compressions without pausing during ventilation.
- Recheck the rhythm after 2 minutes and proceed accordingly.
- If VF/VT recurs, change to the shockable rhythm algorithm.
- If there is doubt as to whether the rhythm is asystole or fine VF, do *not* attempt defibrillation but continue CPR.
- Give further adrenaline 1 mg IV after every 3–5 minutes (alternate loops).

CPR before defibrillation

- In the case of out-of-hospital cardiac arrest attended – but not witnessed – by health-care professionals equipped with manual defibrillators, give CPR for 2 minutes before defibrillating.
- Do not delay defibrillation if an out-of-hospital arrest has been witnessed by a health-care professional.
- Do not delay defibrillation for an in-hospital cardiac arrest.

Adapted from Resuscitation Council (UK) 2005 Guidelines, which can be found at www.resus.org.uk/pages/als.pdf and which you are encouraged to read.

The primary and secondary surveys

In this station, you are going to be asked to assess a patient with a medical emergency or who has suffered severe injury (e.g. from a road traffic accident). What follows is a general outline of the areas that you are going to need to cover.

Primary survey

The quick look

- Inspect the patient.
- Introduce yourself to him. Is he responsive? Try to elicit a response by shouting out his name.

Airway and cervical spine

- Assess the airway for obstruction.
- If necessary, clear and secure the airway. If there is suspicion of a cervical spine injury, use the jaw-thrust technique.
- If there is a suspicion of cervical spine injury, immobilise the cervical spine in a stiff collar. Place sandbags on either side of the head and tape them across the forehead.

Breathing

- Assess breathing: look, listen, feel.
- Expose the chest.
- Note the rate and depth of respiration.
- Look for asymmetries of chest expansion.
- Look for chest injuries.
- Palpate for tracheal deviation. Palpate, percuss, and auscultate the chest. Try to exclude flail segments, pneumothorax, or haemothorax.
- Attach a pulse oximeter.
- If appropriate, ventilate using a bag, mask, and oropharyngeal airway or endotracheal tube.

Circulation and haemorrhage control

- Control any visible haemorrhage by direct pressure.
- Look for clinical signs of shock: assess the pulse, skin colour, capillary refill time, JVP, heart sounds, and blood pressure. Try to exclude cardiac tamponade.
- Attach an ECG monitor.
- Place two large-bore (grey) cannulas into large peripheral veins.
- Take a sample of blood for group and cross-match.
- Start fluid replacement.

Disability (neurological assessment)

- Assess neurological function on the AVPU scale:
  - A   Alert
  - V   Voice elicits a response
  - P   Pain elicits a response
  - U   Unresponsive

- Assess the pupils for size and reactivity.
- Check that all limb extremities can be moved.

Exposure and environmental control

- Remove the patient's remaining clothing and inspect both his front and back. Log-roll him so that his spine remains immobilised.
- Cover him in a blanket.

Secondary survey

Once the patient is stable:

- Take a short, AMPLE history:
  - **A**llergies
  - **M**edications and tetanus immunity
  - **P**revious medical history
  - **L**ast meal
  - **E**vents leading to the injury
- Carry out a head-to-toe physical examination.
- Monitor ECG, BP, oxygen saturation, and core temperature.
- Insert a urinary catheter and, if necessary, a naso-gastric tube.
- Order investigations: full blood count, urea and electrolytes, liver function tests, amylase, glucose, coagulation profile, arterial blood gases, toxicology screen, and X-rays of the lateral cervical spine, chest, and pelvis.
- Encourage questions from the patient and address his concerns.

Management of medical emergencies

Acute asthma

You are called to see a 28 year old man in A&E. The patient is in obvious respiratory distress, and is struggling to speak. The nurse tells you that the patient has a history of asthma. PEFR is 40% of expected, and oxygen saturation is 91%. What is your immediate course of action?

- Assess the severity of the attack by carrying out a brief physical examination, including ABCs.

  A severe attack is indicated by:
  - PEFR <50% of predicted or best
  - respiratory rate >25/min
  - pulse rate of >110 beats/min
  - inability to complete sentences

  A life-threatening attack is suggested by:
  - oxygen saturation <92%
  - silent chest, cyanosis, poor respiratory effort
  - bradycardia, arrhythmia, or hypotension
  - exhaustion, confusion, or coma

- If this is a severe attack, call for senior or specialist help and inform an anaesthetist and the ITU. Begin treatment immediately.
- Sit the patient up and give 100% oxygen through a non-rebreather mask with a reservoir bag.
- Give 5 mg salbutamol and 0.5 mg ipratropium bromide nebulised with oxygen.
- Give a corticosteroid such as hydrocortisone 100 mg IV, and consider adding prednisolone 30–60 mg (if the patient is not too distressed to take tablets).
- Once the patient is stable, carry out investigations including arterial blood gases (ABGs) and a chest X-ray. A life-threatening attack can be confirmed on ABGs by a $PaO_2 > 8$ kPa, a $PaCO_2 > 5$ kPa (due to poor respiratory effort), and a pH < 7.35 (due to CO_2 retention or lactic acidosis from tissue ischaemia). ABGs can also be used to monitor serum electrolytes, particularly K^+ which may be decreased. Chest X-ray is helpful in excluding differentials such as inhalation of a foreign body, pneumothorax, pulmonary oedema, and acute exacerbation of COPD.
- If initial measures fail, add magnesium sulphate 1.2–2 g IV over 20 minutes and give salbutamol nebulisers every 15 minutes.
- Continue monitoring the patient at regular intervals. If he is still not improving, consider aminophylline IV. Discuss with your seniors and with the ITU.

Acute pulmonary oedema

You are called to the ward to see a 55 year old lady with acute shortness of breath. She was admitted with severe diarrhoea and vomiting, and was therefore being aggressively rehydrated. An old ECG suggests left ventricular damage. On physical examination you find a raised JVP, gallop rhythm, and bilateral crackles. What is your immediate course of action?

- Sit the patient up.
- Give 100% oxygen through a non-rebreather mask with a reservoir bag. Care must be taken if the patient has COPD.
- Obtain IV access and attach an ECG monitor. Treat any arrhythmias as appropriate.
- Give GTN spray 2 puffs SL, unless the patient is hypotensive.
- Give diamorphine 2.5–5 mg IV slowly. Care must be taken if the patient has COPD.

- Give frusemide 40–80 mg IV slowly. Note that both diamorphine and frusemide are primarily acting as vasodilators in this context.
- Once the patient has stabilised, further investigations can be carried out such as arterial blood gases, chest X-ray, cardiac enzymes, and U&Es. Continue monitoring the patient at regular intervals.
- Start a nitrate infusion, e.g. isosorbide dinitrate 2–10 mg/h unless the patient is hypotensive. (If systolic BP is < 100 mmHg, treat as cardiogenic shock.)
- If the patient deteriorates, discuss with your seniors and with ITU. Consider increasing the nitrate infusion or giving more frusemide. Re-consider alternative diagnoses such as asthma, COPD, pneumonia, and pulmonary embolism.
- As this patient has left ventricular failure, an ACE-I is indicated once her condition has stabilised.

Acute myocardial infarction

You are tending to a 65 year old gentleman with known cardiovascular disease when he suddenly clutches his chest in severe pain. You look up at the cardiac monitor and see prominent ST elevation. What is your immediate course of action?

- Assess ABCs.
- Give 100% oxygen through a non-rebreather mask with a reservoir bag.
- If not already in place, set up continuous cardiac monitoring and obtain a 12-lead ECG.
- Gain IV access and take blood for baseline troponins, FBC, U&Es, glucose, and lipids.
- If possible, carry out a brief assessment of the patient, including brief history and focused physical examination.
- Give morphine 5–10 mg IV with an antiemetic. Two puffs of GTN SL can be given to provide further relief if the patient is not hypotensive.
- Give aspirin 300 mg PO.
- If the patient is diabetic or the blood glucose is >11 mmol/l, an insulin sliding scale may be indicated.
- For a STEMI, thrombolysis should ideally be given within 90 minutes, e.g. streptokinase 1.5 million units in 100 ml saline IVI over 1 hour. Alteplase may be indicated if the patient has previously received streptokinase. In equipped centres, primary percutaneous coronary angioplasty can be considered in lieu of thrombolysis.

The indications for thrombolysis are:

- ST elevation of >2 mm in 2 or more chest leads
- ST elevation of >1 mm in 2 or more limb leads
- New onset LBBB
- Posterior MI, as evidenced by dominant R waves and ST depression in leads V1–3

Ensure that there are no contraindications to thrombolysis such as internal bleeding or severe liver disease. If so, consider urgent angioplasty instead of thrombolysis.

- Following thrombolysis, give a beta blocker such as atenolol 5 mg IV and an ACE inhibitor such as lisinopril 2.5 mg (unless contraindicated).
- For a NSTEMI, give LMWH, a beta blocker such as atenolol 5 mg IV, and IV nitrates (unless contraindicated). Medium and high risk patients should be given an infusion of GPIIb/IIIa and urgent angiography. Low risk patients may be discharged following a stress test (exercise ECG/stress echo).
- Following an MI, and unless there are any contraindications, the patient should receive:
  - long term low-dose aspirin
  - clopidogrel (4 weeks for STEMI, 3 months for NSTEMI)
  - long term statin

- long term beta blocker
- long term ACE inhibitor

Massive pulmonary embolism

You are fast-bleeped to the ward, where a 48 year old lady who had surgery for ovarian carcinoma 12 days ago has collapsed on the toilet. She has developed acute dyspnoea with pleuritic chest pain. You assess ABCs and carry out a brief physical examination and find tachycardia, hypotension, and signs of right ventricular strain. What is your immediate course of action?

- Give 100% oxygen through a non-rebreather mask with a reservoir bag.
- Obtain IV access. Take blood for FBC, clotting screen, D-dimers, cardiac enzymes, U&Es, and creatinine. ABGs should also be taken and may reveal reduced PaO_2, reduced $PaCO_2$, and acidosis.
- Give morphine 10 mg IV with an anti-emetic.
- Start unfractionated heparin 10 000 U IV bolus, then 18 U/kg/h IVI as guided by APTT. Low molecular weight heparin can be given as an alternative.
- If systolic BP is >90 mmHg, confirm the diagnosis by carrying out ECG, chest X-ray, and computed tomographic pulmonary angiogram (CTPA) which is the gold standard for diagnosing PE. Chest X-ray is most often normal, but is useful in excluding other chest disease such as pneumothorax and pneumonia. ECG may reveal sinus tachycardia or AF, right ventricular strain, RBBB, and, uncommonly, the S_I, Q_{III}, T_{III} pattern: deep S waves in lead I, Q waves in lead III, and inverted T waves in lead III.
- Start warfarin 10 mg OD PO. Stop heparin once INR is in the range 2–3.
- If systolic BP is <90 mmHg, give a rapid colloid infusion and call for senior help. The patient may require inotropic support and thrombolysis. Surgical embolectomy is an alternative if immediately available.

Status epilepticus

You are the duty A&E doctor when a fitting patient is brought in by ambulance. You establish that the fitting started more than 20 minutes ago. What is your immediate course of action?

- Assess ABCs
- Secure the airway.
- Place the patient in the recovery position.
- Give 100% oxygen through a non-rebreather mask with a reservoir bag to prevent cerebral hypoxia from seizure activity. Regular suctioning may also be required.
- Record and monitor blood pressure.
- Obtain IV access.
- Take bloods for ABGs, glucose, U&Es, calcium, magnesium, LFTs, FBC, toxicology screen, and anticonvulsant levels to try to determine the cause of the seizures, e.g. hypoglycaemia, metabolic disturbance, alcohol, drugs, inadequate anticonvulsant dose, cerebral lesion or infection, and, if the patient is pregnant, eclampsia. Pseudo-seizures are a possibility to bear in mind. Obtain some information about the patient, e.g. from an accompanying relative, if at all possible.
- If hypoglycaemia is suspected to be the cause, give 50 ml of 50% dextrose IV. If alcohol is suspected to be the cause, give thiamine 250 mg IV over 10 minutes.
- To stop the seizures, give a benzodiazepine such as lorazepam 4 mg IV slowly or diazepam 10 mg IV/PR. IV benzodiazepines should only be given if resuscitation facilities are available.
- If this measure is unsuccessful, the next step is a phenytoin IV infusion. With a blood pressure and ECG monitor attached, give 15–18 mg/kg, at less than 50 mg/min.
- If this is unsuccessful, call for senior help and for an anaesthetist. General anaesthesia in ITU may be required.

Diabetic ketoacidosis

A 17 year old boy with no previous medical history presents to A&E complaining of vomiting and abdominal pain. When you see him, he appears severely dehydrated and is breathing heavily. You can smell ketones on his breath. What is your immediate course of action?

- Assess ABCs.
- Obtain a rapid blood glucose and urine dipstick for urinary ketones.
- Establish IV access and take blood for laboratory glucose, osmolality, U&Es, HCO_3^-, amylase, FBC, and blood cultures. Obtain an arterial sample for blood gases.
- Give IV fluids. Be careful, as one of the commonest causes of death in DKA (diabetic ketoacidosis) is from cerebral oedema from over-rapid rehydration. One regimen is to give 1 l of normal saline over 30 min followed by 1 l over 1 hour, 1 l over 2 hour, 1 l over 4 hour, and 1 l over 6 hours. Change to 5% dextrose once blood glucose is 10–15 mmol/l.
- Start a sliding scale of insulin via an IVI pump. Add 50 U of Actrapid to 50 ml of saline in a syringe, and give insulin at an initial rate of 4–8 U/h (4–8 ml/h).
- Monitor vital signs, ECG, glucose, U&Es, and HCO_3^-. Aim for a fall in glucose of 5 mmol/h. Plasma K^+ falls as K^+ enters cells, so KCl should be added to IV fluids as appropriate.
- Investigate the cause of the episode and treat any precipitating factors such as infection.
- Other measures:
  - give unfractionated heparin 5000 units TDS SC for venous thromboembolism prophylaxis
  - consider a naso-gastric tube if the patient is nauseated, vomiting, or unconscious
  - consider a urinary catheter if there is persistent hypotension, cardiac failure, renal failure, or no urine output for 2 hours
  - consider a CVP line in the frail and elderly or if there is cardiac failure or renal failure

Acute poisoning

- Carry out ABCs and take action as appropriate. Nurse in semi-prone position if unconscious.
- If possible, take a focussed history from the patient or friends/relatives focussing in particular on:
  - the drugs ingested and their quantities
  - associated alcohol or drug use
  - symptoms, including vomiting
  - other aspects of the history, particularly past medical history, past psychiatric history, and drug history

Carry out a full physical examination. If no history is available, try to identify the ingested drug from your findings.

Table 27. Acute poisoning – identifying the ingested drug	
Drug	**Signs and symptoms**
Paracetamol	Initially: none or nausea, vomiting, and RUQ pain
	Later: jaundice, hypoglycaemia, encephalopathy, renal failure
Salicylates	Vomiting, dehydration, increased respiratory rate, hyperventilation, sweating, warm extremities, bounding pulse, tinnitus, vertigo, deafness, metabolic disturbances, pulmonary oedema, renal failure, seizures, coma
Opiates	Pin-point pupils (sometimes absent if other drugs are involved), nausea, vomiting, drowsiness, respiratory depression, coma

- Obtain IV access and take blood for FBC, U&Es, creatinine, LFTs, INR/PT/clotting screen, blood glucose, paracetamol and salicylate levels, other specific drug levels (as appropriate, contact senior colleagues or the National Poisons Information Service if unsure). Other investigations that need to be carried out include urine/serum toxicology screen, ABGs, and an ECG.
- Monitor vital signs such as respiratory rate, oxygen saturation, pulse rate, blood pressure, and temperature. Consider attaching a cardiac monitor to monitor ECG and inserting a urinary catheter to monitor urinary output.
- If appropriate, consider
  - gastric emptying and lavage, NB: gastric lavage alone is rarely used
  - activated charcoal (50 g in 200 ml water) to reduce the absorption of, for example, paracetamol or salicylates from the gut

Paracetamol

- Specialist help from the gastroenterology team should be sought early if severe liver damage is likely. In adults, 150 mg/kg or more may be fatal.
- Transfer to a specialist unit if systolic BP < 80 mmHg, blood pH < 7.3, INR > 2, creatinine > 200, or there are signs of encephalopathy or increased intracranial pressure.
- Repeat paracetamol level, ideally at 4 hours post-ingestion.

Figure 71. Paracetamol poisoning: normal and high-risk treatment lines.

- If < 8 hours post-ingestion and paracetamol level is above the normal treatment line, give N-acetylcysteine (NAC, Parvolex) IVI as per protocol. If the patient is malnourished (e.g. in anorexia or alcoholism), or on an enzyme-inducing drug, prefer the high-risk treatment line instead (Figure 70).
- If > 8 hours post-ingestion and the patient has taken a significant overdose, start N-acetylcysteine and stop if paracetamol level returns below the treatment line and INR/ALT is normal. Note that paracetamol level is unreliable after 15 hours or in the event of a staggered overdose; simply treat according to the initial amount ingested.
- Continue monitoring vital signs at regular intervals and repeat U&Es, creatinine, LFTs, and INR/PT on the next day.

Salicylates

- IV fluid to correct any dehydration, with particular attention to K+ supplements.
- Give 1.26% sodium bicarbonate IVI to correct any metabolic acidosis.
- Repeat salicylate level at 2 hours post-ingestion: levels above 700 mg/l are potentially fatal: call for senior or specialist help.
- If plasma level > 700 mg/l or severe acidosis, renal failure, heart failure, or seizures, consider haemodialysis.
- Monitor salicylate levels, ABGs, blood glucose, U&Es, and urinary output.

Opiates

- Naloxone, e.g. 0.4–2 mg IV, titrated to response.
- As naloxone has a shorter half-life than opiates, it may need to be given often or as an intravenous infusion to prevent re-occurrence of signs and symptoms. If the patient is threatening to self-discharge, it can be given IM.
- Naloxone may precipitate severe withdrawal in high-dose opiate misusers, who may be very angry at you for ruining their 'trip'.

Once the patient is medically stable, he should be referred for a psychiatric assessment.

Bag-valve mask ventilation

Specifications: A mannequin in lieu of a patient.

- Open the airway using the head-tilt, chin-lift method. Remove any visible obstruction from the mouth.
- Identify the need for a Guedel airway (e.g. if the airway is obstructed or the patient is unconscious).
- Size the Guedel airway by measuring the distance from the incisors to the angle of the jaw. The most commonly used sizes are 2 for a small adult, 3 for a medium adult, and 4 for a large adult.
- Insert the Guedel airway so that its concave side faces away from the tongue. After inserting it almost to the back of the pharynx, rotate it 180 degrees and slide it in to its full extent.
- Choose an appropriately sized bag-valve mask.
- Attach the bag-valve mask to an oxygen supply. Adjust the flow rate to 15 l per minute.
- Hold the mask over the face with your dominant hand. Place your thumb over the nose and support the jaw with the middle and ring fingers (*Figure 72*). Ensuring a tight seal is difficult, so make sure you get sufficient practice.
- Maintain the head-tilt, chin-lift position.
- Use your free hand to compress the bag.
- Look for a rise in the chest.

Figure 72. Bag-valve mask ventilation technique.

 If a second person is available (e.g. the examiner), use both hands to hold the mask and get him to squeeze the bag.

- Ventilate at a rate of 10 compressions per minute until the patient starts breathing or until the patient can be intubated and put on a ventilator.

Station 92

Laryngeal mask insertion

Specifications: A mannequin in lieu of a patient.

Table 28. Laryngeal mask sizes	
Size 1	Infant
Size 2	Child
Size 3	Small adult
Size 4	Normal adult
Size 5	Large adult

The equipment

Gather in a tray:

- A pair of non-sterile gloves.
- Laryngeal mask of appropriate size (see *Table 28*).
- Lubricant.
- An air-filled syringe.
- A bandage.

Before inserting the laryngeal mask

- Don the gloves.
- Assemble the equipment.
- Check inflation and deflation of the laryngeal mask.
- Lubricate the laryngeal mask.
- Ensure that the patient has received adequate anaesthesia (the cough reflex should be suppressed).
- Ensure that the patient has been pre-oxygenated, or pre-oxygenate him by bag ventilation for 1 minute.
- Use the head-tilt, chin-lift technique to ensure that the mouth is fully open.
- Check the state of the dentition.

Inserting the laryngeal mask

- Insert the tip of the mask into the mouth, ensuring that the aperture is facing the tongue.
- Press the tip of the mask against the hard palate as you introduce it into the pharynx.
- Use your index finger to guide the tube into the pharynx until resistance can be felt.
- Check that the black line on the tube is facing the upper lip.

 If you do not succeed in inserting the laryngeal mask within 30 seconds, you must pre-oxygenate the patient a second time before you try again.

Epiglottis
Larynx
Cuff
Trachea
Oesophagus

Figure 73. Laryngeal mask insertion.

After inserting the laryngeal mask

- Inflate the cuff, ensuring that you do not over-inflate it. A size 3 mask needs <20 ml of air, a size 4 <30 ml, and a size 5 <40 ml.
- Secure the cuff in place by means of a length of bandage.
- Attach the breathing system and check that the patient is being satisfactorily ventilated.

Pre-operative assessment

The surgical pre-assessment is about half the job of a surgical house officer, so is not unlikely to be examined in a final year OSCE. The aims of the pre-operative assessment are primarily to:

- Ascertain that the patient is fit for surgery and anaesthesia.
- Take appropriate action if he is not.
- Ensure that he fully understands the proposed procedure.
- Ensure that he fully understands the peri-operative process and any special requirements of the proposed procedure.
- Minimise any remaining fears or anxieties.

[Note] The responsibility for gaining informed consent from the patient is no longer that of the junior house officer, but that of the operating surgeon.

Specifications: In this station you may be asked to talk through or carry out a part or parts of the pre-operative assessment.

Before starting

- Introduce yourself to the patient.
- Explain that you are going to ask him some questions and carry out a physical examination to assess his fitness for surgery.
- Ensure that he is comfortable.

The assessment

History

- Medical history, in particular:
  - previous surgery and anaesthesia – ask specifically about history of anaesthetic complications, e.g. suxamethonium apnoea, malignant hyperpyrexia
  - previous hospital admissions
  - cardiovascular: hypertension, palpitations, angina, myocardial infarction, cardiac failure, orthopnoea, other 'heart problems', stroke or TIA
  - respiratory: dyspnoea, asthma, cough, tuberculosis
  - GI and renal: dysphagia, heartburn, liver disease, renal failure
  - other: diabetes, sickle cell anaemia, epilepsy, neuromuscular problems
- Drug history:
  - prescribed medication – ask specifically about recent changes in medication, insulin, and anticoagulants
  - over-the-counter and alternative medication
  - recreational drugs (especially cocaine, ecstasy, and narcotics)
- Allergies including to antiseptic, plaster, and latex.
- Smoking.
- Alcohol.

[Note] Most drugs should be taken as normal on the day of the surgery, although special advice is needed for insulin and anticoagulants.

- Family history of allergic reactions, anaesthetic complications, medical and surgical conditions.
- Social history, e.g. level of support in post-operative period.

Physical examination

- Record height and weight and calculate his body mass index as given by weight in kilograms/(height in metres)^2, e.g. 70 kg/(1.8 m)^2 = 21.6 (normal 20–25).
- Examine the cardiovascular, respiratory, gastrointestinal, and neurological systems.
- Assess neck mobility by asking the patient to flex and extend his neck.
- Assess jaw mobility by asking the patient to open and close his mouth.
- Inspect the state of the dentition.
- Carry out a Mallampati pharyngeal assessment. To do this you need to ask the patient to open his mouth as wide as possible and to extend his tongue (*Figure 74*).

I	II	III	IV

Figure 74. Mallampati pharyngeal assessment:
  I – Pharyngeal pillars, soft palate, and uvula visible;
  II – Soft palate and uvula visible;
  III – Soft palate and the base of the uvula visible;
  IV – Soft palate not visible
  NB: Mallampati scores of III or IV are relative contraindications to surgery

- Determine the ASA physical status rating, a health index at the time of surgery (*Table 29*).

Table 29. The ASA physical status rating	
1*	Healthy, no systemic disturbance
2*	Mild/moderate systemic disease. No activity limitation.
3*	Severe systemic disturbance. Some activity limitation.
4*	Life-threatening systemic disturbance. Severe activity limitation.
5*	Moribund with limited chance of survival.
* Add suffix *E* for emergency.	

Pre-operative investigations

Table 30. Indications for pre-operative investigations	
Group and save/cross-match	Group and save for e.g. cholecystectomy, ERCP, mastectomy, amputation
	Cross-match for e.g. laparotomy (2 units), TURP (3 units), hip replacement (4 units), liver surgery (6 units), aneurysm repair (4 units if elective, 10 units if emergency)
FBC	Cardiorespiratory disease, anaemia, blood loss, chronic disease, blood disorders, on an oral anticoagulant, alcohol misuse, female patients, male patients > 40 years
Clotting screen	Liver disease, alcohol misuse, on an anticoagulant
Sickle cell screening	Patients from Africa, the Caribbean, and the Mediterranean
U&Es	Hypertension, heart failure, renal failure, liver disease, diabetes, dehydration, starvation, on diuretics, digoxin, steroids, or lithium, age > 60 and having major surgery
Glucose	Diabetes, obesity, on steroids
LFTs (including clotting screen)	Liver disease, alcohol misuse, malignancy, malnutrition
ECG	Arrhythmias, angina, myocardial infarction, heart murmurs, heart failure, cardiovascular risk factors, age > 50
CXR	Hypertension, cardiorespiratory disease or symptoms, malignancy, > 60 years old and having major surgery, recent immigrant
Cervical spine X-ray	Severe chronic rheumatoid arthritis, cervical spondylosis
Other	TFTs in thyroid disease
	Amylase in abdominal pain or hepatobiliary surgery
	Lung function tests in severe respiratory disease
	Drug levels, e.g. if on digoxin or lithium
	HIV

Peri-operative management

Explain about:

- Fasting, in most cases:
    - stop solids from 6 hours before the operation
    - stop milky drinks from 4 hours
    - stop clear fluids (and chewing gum) from 2 hours
- Pre-medication:
    - benzodiazepines can be given before the operation to help the patient feel sleepy or less anxious
- The anaesthetic procedure:
    - patient information about different anaesthetic procedures can be obtained from www.kch.nhs.uk/patients/general-information/leaflets/ – look for "You and Your Anaesthetic"
- Post-operative pain relief:
    - oral analgesia, e.g. paracetamol, cocodamol, NSAIDs such as diclofenac and ibuprofen, tramadol, opiates
    - parenteral analgesia
    - suppositories

- local anaesthetics and regional blocks
- patient-controlled analgesia
- patches
- Post-operative nausea and vomiting:
  - explain to the patient that he may feel sick after the operation and reassure him that this is quite normal and that he can be given an anti-sickness tablet or injection
- Going home and driving.

After the procedure

- Ask the patient if he has any remaining questions or concerns.
- Thank the patient.
- Order the appropriate investigations (*Table 30*) and remember to check up on the results!
- Talk to the anaesthetist if you have any concerns.

Syringe driver operation

There are two different sorts of syringe driver: the 50 ml syringe pump, frequently used for heparin, glyceryl trinitrate, and insulin infusions, and for epidural and patient-controlled analgesia; and the Graseby syringe driver, which installs a 10 ml or 20 ml syringe and is frequently used in palliative care. There are two varieties of the Graseby syringe driver: the blue Graseby MS 16A, which is designed to be programmed at an hourly rate, and the green Graseby MS 26, which is designed to be programmed at a 12, 24, or 48 hourly rate. In this station, you may be required to set up and operate a Graseby syringe driver for two drugs, e.g. diamorphine and cyclizine.

Figure 75. The blue Graseby MS 16A, designed to be programmed at an hourly rate.

Before starting

- Introduce yourself to the patient.
- Explain the need for a syringe driver and the procedure involved, and gain consent.
- Gather the appropriate equipment.

The equipment

- Non-sterile gloves.
- Graseby syringe driver (check the battery is in place and the device is functioning).
- Luer-lock syringe (10 ml or 20 ml).
- Subcutaneous giving set.
- Drug.
- Diluent (sterile water or normal saline).

Emergency medicine and anaesthesiology

The procedure

- Consult the prescription chart and check:
  - the identity of the patient
  - the prescription: drug(s), dose(s), diluent, route of administration, duration of the infusion, date and time of starting
  - drug allergies
- Check the name, dose, and expiry date of the drug(s) on the vial(s).
- Ask a colleague (registered nurse or doctor) to confirm the name, dose, and expiry date of the drug(s) on the vial(s).
- Don a pair of non-sterile gloves.
- Draw up the correct doses of the drugs into the Luer-lock syringe.
- Draw up the correct diluent to make up the requested volume (stated on the prescription chart) and shake the syringe with the needle capped.
- Connect the giving set to the syringe and run the infusion through it.
- Calculate the rate of infusion by measuring the length of liquid in the syringe in millimetres and dividing it by the number of hours (Graseby 16A) or days (Graseby MS 26) over which the infusion should be given.
- Label the syringe with:
  - the patient's name, date of birth, and hospital number
  - the date and time of preparation
  - drugs used and their doses
  - diluent used and its volume
  - rate of infusion
  - your name
- Place the syringe into the syringe driver and secure the device.
- Set the syringe driver to the rate required.
- Place the giving set subcutaneously and start the infusion.

After the procedure

- Sign the drug chart, and have your checking colleague countersign it.
- Ask the patient if he has any questions or concerns.
- Ensure that he is comfortable.

Patient-Controlled Analgesia (PCA) explanation

In PCA, the patient presses a button to activate an infusion pump and receive a pre-prescribed intravenous bolus of analgesic, most commonly morphine or another opioid such as diamorphine, pethidine, or fentanyl.

Advantages

- Prevents delays in analgesic administration and thereby minimises pain. In the post-operative period this may forestall a number of adverse events such as disability, pressure sores, DVT, PE, atelectasis, and constipation.
- Minimises the amount of analgesic used, as the patient only activates the pump if he is actually in pain. Other people, such as relatives, should be told not to activate the pump.
- Provides a reliable indication of the patient's pain, and its evolution over time.
- Reduces the chance of dangerous medication errors, as the pump is programmed according to a set prescription and 'locks out' if the patient tries to activate it too often. A typical dose regimen is a 0.5–2.0 mg bolus of morphine with a lock-out of 10–15 minutes.

Disadvantages

- Patients may not receive enough analgesia (see later). In particular, patients may wake up in pain, as they cannot press the button when they are asleep.
- Patients may be physically or mentally unable to press a button.
- The pumps are expensive and may malfunction, especially if the battery is not adequately charged.

Side-effects

Side-effects of morphine include:

- respiratory depression
- sedation
- nausea and vomiting
- constipation
- urinary retention
- pruritus

Some of these side-effects can be controlled by additional prescriptions of, for example, anti-emetics, laxatives, or antihistamines. If the patient is suffering from significant respiratory depression or sedation, the dose should be decreased and alternative analgesia considered. (Remember that respiratory depression or sedation can also be caused by important post-operative complications, so do not omit to exclude these.)

Monitoring

Patients should be reviewed at regular intervals for pain, analgesic usage, and side-effects; observations should be made of the patient's pain score, analgesic usage, pulse, blood pressure, respiratory rate, and oxygen saturation. If pain relief is inadequate, the dose regime should be altered. In some cases, a continuous 'background' infusion might be considered.

Epidural analgesia explanation

Epidural analgesia, or 'epidural', is a form of regional anaesthesia involving the injection of local anaesthetics and/or opioids through a catheter inserted into the epidural space. Epidurals can be indicated for analgesia in labour (often simply as a matter of patient choice), for surgical anaesthesia in certain operations, e.g. caesarean section, and as an adjunct to general anaesthesia in others, e.g. laparatomy, hysterectomy, hip replacement. They can also be indicated for post-operative analgesia, back pain, and palliative care.

Advantages

- Permits analgesia to be delivered as a continuous infusion and/or to be patient-controlled.
- Effective and safe, with a mortality of only about 1 in 100 000.
- In post-operative analgesia, reduces the risk of certain post-operative complications such as nausea and vomiting, chest infections, and constipation.

Disadvantages

- 5% failure rate.
- In labour, increases the risk of an assisted delivery.

Contraindications

Absolute

- Raised intracranial pressure.
- Coagulopathy/anticoagulation.
- Hypovolaemia.
- Skin infection at epidural site.
- Septicaemia.

Relative

- Un-cooperative patient.
- Anatomical abnormalities or previous spinal surgery.
- Certain neurological disorders.
- Certain heart-valve problems.

Procedure

Epidurals are normally performed by a trained anaesthetist with the patient either in the preferred sitting position or in the left lateral position. The planned entry site is identified and marked. After the skin is cleaned and local anaesthetic administered, a Tuohy needle is advanced until a loss of resistance is felt anterior to the *ligamentum flavum*. The cathether, a fine plastic tube, is then threaded through the needle and the needle is removed, leaving the catheter in place. As epidurals are usually carried out in the mid-lumbar region, there is very little risk of injuring the spinal cord.

Figure 76. Anatomy of the epidural space.

Side-effects and complications

- Side-effects of opioids.
- In higher doses can result in loss of other modalities of sensation (such as touch and proprioception) and motor function.
- Hypotension, most often resulting from loss of sympathetic function.
- Urinary retention.
- Accidental dural puncture resulting in a leak and a severe headache that is exacerbated by raising the head above horizontal.
- Accidental infusion into the CSF resulting in a high block or, more rarely, a total spinal involving profound hypotension, respiratory paralysis, and unconsciousness.
- Epidural haematoma that can cause spinal compression.
- Abscess formation.

Monitoring

Patients receiving epidural analgesia should be monitored for pain intensity, drug-related side-effects, and signs of complications due to the epidural procedure.

Wound suturing

Specifications: A pad of 'skin' in lieu of a patient. This station most likely requires you to talk through the parts of the procedure and then to demonstrate your suturing technique. For this second part, there can be no substitute for practice, practice, and more practice!

Before starting

- Introduce yourself to the patient.
- Explain the procedure and ask for his consent to carry it out.
- Examine the wound, looking for debris, dirt, and tendon damage.
- Indicate that you would request an X-ray to exclude a foreign body.
- Assess distal motor, sensory, and vascular function.
- Position the patient appropriately and ensure that he is comfortable.

The equipment

Gather in a tray or on a trolley:

- a pair of non-sterile gloves
- a suture pack
- a suture of appropriate type and size (natural/synthetic, absorbable/non-absorbable)
- a 5 ml syringe, 21G and 25G needles, and a vial of local anaesthetic (e.g. 1% lignocaine)
- antiseptic solution
- a sharps bin

The procedure

- Wash your hands.
- Open the suture pack, thus creating a sterile field.
- Pour antiseptic solution into the receptacle.
- Open the suture, the syringe, and both needles onto the sterile field.
- Wash your hands using sterile technique.
- Don the non-sterile gloves.
- Attach a 21G needle to the syringe.
- Ask an assistant (the examiner) to open the vial of local anaesthetic and draw up 5 ml of local anaesthetic. For an average 70 kg adult, up to 20 ml of 1% lignocaine can be safely used, although 5–10 ml is usually sufficient. Epinephrine may be used with lignocaine to minimise bleeding. The maximum safe dose of lignocaine with or without epinephrine is 7 mg/kg and 3 mg/kg respectively. However, avoid injecting epinephrine when anaesthetising the extremities due to the risk of ischaemic tissue necrosis.
- Discard the needle into the sharps bin and attach the 25G needle to the syringe.
- Clean the wound (use forceps) with antiseptic-soaked cotton wool and drape the field. Dirty wounds may benefit from cleansing with povidone iodine, whereas normal saline can be used to cleanse and irrigate 'clean' wounds.
- Inject the local anaesthetic into the apices and edges of the wound. Make sure to pull back on the plunger before injecting.
- Discard the needle into the sharps bin.
- Indicate that you would give the anaesthetic 5–10 minutes to operate (or as long as it takes).

- Apply the sutures approximately 3 mm from the wound edge and 5–10 mm apart. Use needle-holding forceps to hold the needle and toothed forceps to pick up the skin margins. Knot the sutures around the needle-holding forceps.

Figure 77. Use needle-holding forceps to hold the needle approximately two-thirds from the needle tip.

Figure 78. Suggested approach for suturing. Knot the sutures around the needle-holding forceps: loop the suture twice around the nose of the needle-holding forceps using your hand. Then take hold of the short end of the suture with the needle-holding forceps and carry it through the loops, gently pulling the knot tight. Two further single loops are then added in a similar fashion to secure the knot. Each loop is pulled in the opposite direction across the wound edge.

After the procedure

- Clean the wound and indicate that you would apply a dressing.
- Assess the need for a tetanus injection.

- Give appropriate instructions for wound care and indicate the date sutures should be removed (e.g. face 3–4 days, scalp 5 days, trunk 7 days, arm or leg 7–10 days, foot 10–14 days).
- Ask if the patient has any questions or concerns.
- Thank the patient.

Blood glucose measurement and interpretation

Specifications: In this station you are far more likely to be asked to talk through the procedure rather than carry it out on a patient or actor.

Before starting

- Introduce yourself to the patient.
- Explain the procedure and ask for his consent to carry it out.
- Establish when he last ate (fasting blood glucose is usually carried out in the morning before the patient has had anything to eat or drink).

The equipment

In a tray, gather:

- A pair of gloves.
- An alcohol wipe.
- A glucose monitor.
- Test strips.

- A spring-loaded pricker.
- A lancet.
- Cotton wool.

The procedure

- Ask the patient to wash and dry his hands, or use an alcohol wipe to clean the finger that you are going to prick.
- Massage the finger from its base to its tip to increase its perfusion.
- Turn on the glucose monitor and ensure that it is calibrated.
- Check that the test strips have not expired.
- Insert a test strip into the glucose monitor.
- Load the lancet into the pricker and prick the side of the finger.

 It is less painful to prick the side rather than the tip of a finger because there are comparatively fewer nerve endings there.

- Squeeze the finger to obtain a droplet of blood. If no or insufficient blood is obtained, prick the finger again. If this happens, be sympathetic to the patient's plight.
- Place the droplet of blood on the test strip, so as to cover the sensor entirely.
- Give the patient some cotton wool to stop any bleeding.
- Record the reading on the monitor. Units are in millimoles per litre.

After the procedure

- Tell that patient their blood glucose and explain its significance and any further action that needs to be taken, e.g. fasting blood glucose, glucose tolerance test, laboratory measurement. Note that the diagnosis of diabetes in a symptomatic patient should never be made on the basis of a single abnormal blood glucose measurement.
- Ask the patient if he has any questions or concerns.
- Thank the patient.

Table 31. Blood glucose measurement: interpretation of result (normal results vary from lab to lab)	
	Units are in millimoles per litre
Normal	
fasting glucose	< 6.0
non-fasting glucose*	< 7.8
Impaired glucose tolerance	
fasting glucose	6–7
non-fasting glucose	7.8–11.1
Diabetes mellitus	
fasting glucose	≥ 7.0
non-fasting glucose	≥ 11.1
* 2-h post 75 g glucose.	

Examiner's questions

Complications of type II diabetes

Hyperosmolar non-ketotic coma (HONK), retinopathy and cataracts, nephropathy progressing to renal failure, cardiovascular disease predisposing to increased risk of myocardial infarction and stroke, peripheral vascular disease, peripheral and autonomic neuropathy (most frequently distal symmetric sensorimotor polyneuropathy in a glove-and-stocking distribution and oculomotor mononeuropathy), infections, foot ulcers progressing to diabetic foot disease, impotence, miscarriage, stillbirth.

Figure 79. Diabetic foot.

Reproduced from www.londonvascularclinic.com with permission.

Station 99

Urine sample testing and interpretation

Before starting

- Introduce yourself to the patient.
- Take a very brief history from him.
- Explain that you are going to test his urine and explain why.
- Ensure that the urine specimen is fresh and that it has been appropriately collected.

The equipment

- Urine dipstick and urine dipstick bottle.
- A pair of gloves.
- A pen and paper (or the patient's case notes).

The procedure

- Put on the gloves.
- Check that the urine is a mid-stream sample.
- Inspect the colour and appearance of the urine.
- Stir the urine bottle to ensure that the urine is mixed.
- Check the expiry date on the urine dipstick jar.
- Briefly immerse the urine dipstick into the urine specimen.
- Tap off any excess urine from the dipstick.
- Hold the strip horizontally.
- After 2 minutes, read each colour pad using the colour chart on the dipstick bottle.
- Report and record the results.
- Discard the used urine dipstick and the gloves.
- Wash your hands.

Figure 80. The colour chart on the urine dipstick bottle.

After testing the urine

- Explain the results to the patient.
- Document the results in the patient's notes.
- If abnormal, suggest obtaining a second sample of urine or sending the urine for laboratory analysis.
- Thank the patient.

Table 32. Urine dipstick: interpretation of results	
Leukocytes	Urinary tract infection
Nitrites	Bacteriuria, contaminated sample
Protein	Kidney damage or disease, standing upright for prolonged periods, exercise, fever, pregnancy, rarer causes, e.g. leukaemia, multiple myeloma, pre-eclampsia
Blood	Kidney damage or disease, urinary calculi, urinary tract infection, contaminated sample, exercise, dehydration, myoglobinuria
Ketones	Diabetic ketoacidosis, starvation, alcohol intoxication
Glucose	Diabetes mellitus, pregnancy

Station 100

Blood test interpretation

1. Reference ranges are based on a Gaussian or normal distribution, and usually include about 95% of the population. This means that a result only slightly outside the reference range is not necessarily 'abnormal'.
2. Reference ranges do vary from one laboratory to another – don't let this confuse you!

Full blood count

	Normal range
Hb	13–18 g/dl (males); 11.5–16 g/dl (females)
RCC	$4.5–6.5 \times 10^{12}/l$ (males); $3.9–5.6 \times 10^{12}/l$ (females)
PCV	0.4–0.54 (males); 0.37–0.47 (females)
MCV	76–96 fl
MCHC	30–36 g/dl
WCC	$4.0–11.0 \times 10^9/l$
neutrophils	$2.0–7.5 \times 10^9/l$ (40–75% WCC)
lymphocytes	$1.3–3.5 \times 10^9/l$ (20–45%)
eosinophils	$0.04–0.44 \times 10^9/l$ (1–6%)
basophils	$0–0.10 \times 10^9/l$ (0–1%)
monocytes	$0.2–0.8 \times 10^9/l$ (2–10%)
Platelets	$150–400 \times 10^9/l$

- Haemoglobin (Hb) and red cell count (RCC) are increased in dehydration, chronic hypoxia, or polycythaemia. The term 'anaemia' describes a Hb of < 13 g/dl in males and < 11.5 g/dl in females. Anaemia has many causes, including iron deficiency, folate or vitamin B12 deficiency, chronic illness, blood loss, and blood cell destruction.
- Packed cell volume (PCV) or 'haematocrit' is the fraction of total blood volume occupied by red cells; it decreases in anaemia and increases in dehydration, chronic hypoxia, and polycythaemia.
- Mean corpuscular volume (MCV) is the average volume of a red blood cell, and is thus equivalent to PCV/RCC; it decreases in iron deficiency, chronic disease, thalassaemia, and sideroblastic anaemia and increases in folate or vitamin B12 deficiency, alcoholism, liver disease, hypothyroidism, pregnancy, reticulocytosis (e.g. in haemolysis), and other haematological diseases.
- Mean corpuscular haemoglobin concentration (MCHC) is the average concentration of haemoglobin in red cells, and decreases in iron deficiency, chronic disease, and chronic blood loss.
- A raised white cell count (WCC) or leukocytosis may indicate infection, inflammation, major tissue damage, or certain lymphoproliferative disorders. The *differential* white cell count is useful in determining the probable cause of a leukocytosis. For example, a raised neutrophil count or neutrophilia may indicate acute bacterial infection, acute inflammation, or major tissue damage, and a raised eosinophil count or eosinophilia may indicate an allergic reaction or parasitic infection.
- A raised platelet count or thrombocytosis may result from haemorrhage, chronic inflammatory conditions, hyposplenism, and certain myeloproliferative disorders, e.g. chronic myelogenous leukaemia. A low platelet count or thrombocytopaenia may result from decreased

platelet production (e.g. folate or vitamin B12 deficiency, infection, cancer treatment), increased platelet destruction (e.g. immune thrombocytopaenic purpura, disseminated intravascular coagulation, systemic lupus erythematosus), or certain drugs.

Iron studies (haematinics)

	Normal range
Serum iron	14–31 µmol/l (males); 11–30 µmol/l (females)
Ferritin	12–200 µg/l
TIBC	54–75 µg/l
Folate	2.1 µg/l
Vitamin B12	0.13–0.68 nmol/l

- Ferritin is the main protein that stores iron, and so serum ferritin reflects the body's iron stores.
- Total iron binding capacity (TIBC) reflects the amount of transferrin, a protein that transfers iron from the gut, in the serum.
- Iron deficiency and chronic disease may both lead to a decrease in serum iron, and therefore to a microcytic anaemia. In investigating the cause of a microcytic anaemia, serum iron must be looked at in conjuction with serum ferritin and TIBC. In iron deficiency anaemia, serum ferritin is decreased and TIBC is increased. In contrast, in anaemia of chronic disease, serum ferritin is often increased and TIBC often decreased. Note that, in some cases, anaemic of chronic disease can also present with a normal MCV. Other causes of a normocytic anaemia include acute blood loss and renal failure.
- By contrast, folate and vitamin B12 deficiency result in a macrocytic anaemia. Folate levels decrease if dietary intake of folate is inadequate or if demand for folate is increased (e.g. pregnancy, increased cell turnover) and in alcoholism, malabsorption, pernicious anaemia, and treatment with certain drugs such as phenytoin and sodium valproate. Vitamin B12 levels decrease if dietary intake of vitamin B12 is inadequate, and in malabsorption and pernicious anaemia.

Coagulation tests

	Normal range
PT	10–14 s
APTT	35–45 s
TT	10–15 s
INR	0.9–1.2
D-dimers	<0.5 mg/l

- A lack of factors I, II, V, VII, and X or fibrinogen leads to an increase in prothrombin time (PT). PT thus tests the extrinsic system and is prolonged by warfarin treatment, vitamin K deficiency, liver disease, and DIC.
- A lack of factors I, II, V, VIII, IX, XI, or XII leads to an increase in activated partial thromboplastin time (APTT). APTT thus tests the intrinsic system and is prolonged by heparin treatment, haemophilia, liver disease, and DIC.
- Thrombin time (TT) is prolonged by a deficiency of factor I (fibrinogen), heparin treatment, and DIC.
- INR is the ratio of PT to mean PT in a normal population, and should thus be around 1. Target

INR for DVT and PE prophylaxis is 2–3 (3.5 if recurrent), but 3–4 for prosthetic metallic heart valves.
- D-dimers are a fibrin degradation product, and are raised in DVT, PE, and DIC, but also in inflammatory states.

ESR

	Normal range
ESR	< 20 mm/h
	Or, for males, (age in years)/2, and for females (age in years + 10)/2

- A raised erythrocyte sedimentation rate (ESR) is a non-specific finding that often results from inflammation, but sometimes also from injury or malignancy. Serial ESR measurements can be used to monitor disease severity and treatment response in inflammatory disorders such as rheumatoid arthritis and temporal arteritis.

Thyroid function tests

	Normal range
TSH	0.5–5.7 mU/l
Thyroxine (T4)	70–140 nmol/l
Free T4	9–22 pmol/l
Tri-iodothyronine (T3)	1.2–3 nmol/l
TBG	7–17 mg/l

- Typical findings in hyperthyroidism are decreased TSH (thyroid-stimulating hormone) and increased (or normal) T4, free T4, and T3.
- Typical findings in hypothyroidism are increased TSH and decreased (or normal) T4 and free T4.
- Increased TSH and increased T4 suggest a TSH-secreting tumour.
- Decreased TSH, T4, and T3 suggest pituitary disease or 'sick euthyroidism', which can be seen in any systemic illness.
- T4 and T3 are increased if TBG (thyroxine-binding globulin) is increased (e.g. in pregnancy or oestrogen therapy) and vice versa.

Liver function tests

	Normal range
Bilirubin	3–17 µmol/l
ALT	5–35 U/l
AST	5–35 U/l
ALP	30–150 U/l
GGT	11–51 U/l (males); 7–33 U/l (females)
Albumin	35–50 g/l

- The amount of bilirubin in the blood reflects the balance between that produced by red cell destruction and that removed by the liver. A raised bilirubin level results either from diseases causing increased red blood cell destruction, diseases causing hepatocellular damage, or diseases causing biliary obstruction and thereby restricting the excretion of bilirubin. The latter is suggested by a high ratio of conjugated bilirubin to unconjugated bilirubin.
- Raised ALT and AST suggest hepatocellular damage. ALT (alanine aminotransferase) is a relatively specific marker of hepatocellular damage, and is most raised in the acute phase. Although ALT is also present in cardiac muscle, the rises seen in myocardial infarction are comparatively small. AST is a less specific marker of hepatocellular damage than ALT and may also be raised in myocardial infarction, skeletal muscle damage, haemolysis, shock, pregnancy, and exercise.
- Raised ALP and GGT suggest biliary obstruction. ALP (alkaline phosphatise) is raised in biliary obstruction, hepatocellular damage, some bone diseases, and pregnancy. GGT (gamma-glutamyl transferase) is raised in alcohol consumption, and also in biliary obstruction and hepatocellular damage.
- Albumin is a genuine test of liver function and falls in chronic liver disease. Other causes for a fall in albumin include malnutrition, malabsorption, nephrotic syndrome, burns, pregnancy, and overhydration, e.g. with IV fluids. A rise in albumin is usually the consequence of dehydration.

Urea and electrolytes

	Normal range
Sodium	135–145 mmol/l
Potassium	3.5–5.0 mmol/l
Calcium (total)	2.12–2.65 mmol/l
Bicarbonate	24–28 mmol/l
Urea	2.5–6.7 mmol/l
Creatinine	70–150 µmol/l

Hyponatraemia

- Hyponatraemia is commonly caused by the syndrome of inappropriate secretion of anti-diuretic hormone (SIADH), which itself has a large number of causes including malignancy, pulmonary disorders, central nervous system disorders, and drugs. Other common causes of hyponatraemia are inappropriate fluid therapy, diuretic treatment, diarrhoea and vomiting, and cardiac and renal failure. For the causes of hyponatraemia, see Figure 81. Note that high serum glucose, urea, proteins, or lipids can increase serum volume and result in a pseudohyponatraemia.
- Hyponatraemia may be asymptomatic or may produce nausea, vomiting, headache, confusion, convulsions, and coma.
- Treat the cause. It is important to determine the volume status of the patient. If the patient is hypovolaemic, a normal saline infusion may be indicated. Particularly in chronic hyponatraemia, correction should be cautious and gradual (a maximum of 15 mmol/day) so as to avoid the complication of central pontine myelinosis. If the patient is hypervolaemic, fluid restriction (with or without frusemide) may be indicated. Hypertonic saline should only be used in emergency situations.

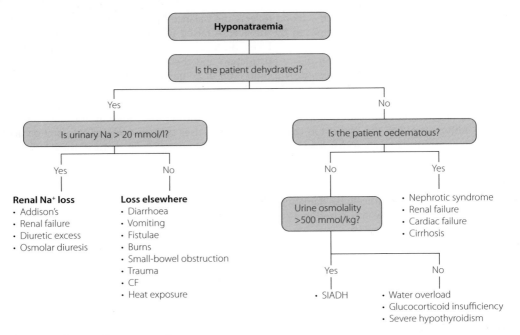

Figure 81. Causes of hyponatraemia.

Hypernatraemia

- Causes include:
  - insufficient water intake
  - inappropriate fluid therapy
  - fluid loss, e.g. through diarrhoea, vomiting, and burns
  - diuretic treatment
  - osmotic diuresis, e.g. in hyperglycaemia
  - diabetes insipidus
  - mineralocorticoid excess as in Conn's syndrome or Cushing's syndrome
- Symptoms include thirst, confusion, convulsions, and coma.
- Treat through oral rehydration or a 5% dextrose infusion, e.g. 4 litres over 24 hours. Note that over-rapid correction of hypernatraemia can lead to cerebral oedema and convulsions, brain damage, and death.

Hypokalaemia

- Causes include:
  - gastrointestinal losses as in vomiting, diarrhoea, laxative use, villous adenoma
  - renal losses as in thiazide or loop diuretic treatment (most common cause), mineralo-corticoid excess (e.g. Conn's syndrome, Cushing's syndrome), and renal tubular acidosis
  - shift into cells as in insulin treatment, metabolic alkalosis, high catecholamines (e.g. due to pain)
  - poor intake as in prolonged fasting, eating disorders
  - re-feeding syndrome
  - hypomagnesaemia

- In mild cases, hypokalaemia is often asymptomic. In severe cases, the clinical picture is dominated by muscle weakness which can progress to flaccid paralysis and, rarely, respiratory failure. ECG changes may include T wave flattening, ST segment depression, appearance of U waves, and tachyarrhythmias.
- Treatment involves addressing the cause and supplementing potassium, either orally or as an intravenous infusion, depending on severity. Note that too concentrated an infusion is painful and damages peripheral veins, and too fast an infusion predisposes to ventricular tachyarrhythmias.

Hyperkalaemia

- Causes include:
  - artefact due to haemolysis of the blood sample (repeat the measurement)
  - excessive intake, most likely in the form of potassium supplements
  - impaired excretion as in renal insufficiency, Addison's disease (reduced mineralocorticoids), treatment with potassium-sparing diuretics and NSAIDs
  - shift out of cells as in diabetic ketoacidosis and other metabolic acidoses
  - excessive release from cells, as in burns, rhabdomyolysis, tumour lysis, massive blood transfusion
- Although hyperkalaemia is usually asymptomatic, it can lead to cardiac arrhythmia and sudden death. For this reason, an ECG should be carried out as soon as hyperkalaemia is suggested. ECG findings include tall, tented T waves, broadened QRS complex, prolonged PR interval, P wave flattening, and a sine wave appearance.
- In mild hyperkalaemia, potassium intake should be restricted. In severe hyperkalaemia, or if there are ECG changes, IV calcium gluconate should be administered to stabilise the myocardium. IV insulin with glucose, the potassium-binding resin calcium resonium, and dialysis can then be used to reduce potassium.

Calcium

- Calcium (total) needs to be adjusted for albumin by adding 0.1 mmol/l for every 4 g/l that albumin is below 40 g/l, and subtracting 0.1 mmol/l for every 4 g/l that albumin is above 40 g/l.
- Hypocalcaemia may be caused by hypomagnesaemia, hyperphosphataemia, hypoparathyroidism, pseudohypoparathyroidism (failure of cells to respond to parathyroid hormone), vitamin D deficiency, and chronic renal failure. Symptoms include depression, perioral paraesthesiae, carpo-pedal spasm (hence Trousseau's sign), neuromuscular excitability (hence Chvostek's sign), tetany, laryngospasm, and cardiac arrhythmias. Treatment involves treating the cause and, depending on severity, oral or IV calcium replacement.
- 90% of cases of hypercalcaemia are accounted for by either malignancy or hyperparathyroidism. Symptoms include fatigue, confusion, depression, anorexia, nausea and vomiting, constipation, abdominal pain, polyuria, renal calculi, and cardiac arrest. Management involves treating the hypercalcaemia and its underlying cause. Treating the hypercalcaemia involves fluids (normal saline), frusemide, and bisphonates, e.g. pamidronate.

For acid–base disturbances, see Station 101.

Urea and creatinine

- Urea is increased in renal disease, renal hypoperfusion (e.g. in severe dehydration), and urinary tract obstruction. It is also increased by a high-protein diet, bleeding into the GI tract, tissue damage, and certain drugs. It is decreased in overhydration, advanced liver disease, malnutrition, and eating disorders.

- Serum creatinine provides a crude estimate of glomerular filtration. It is increased in renal disease, renal hypoperfusion, urinary tract obstruction, and rhabdomyolysis. It is decreased in advanced liver disease, malnutrition, eating disorders, and muscle loss. A better estimate of glomerular filtration is creatinine clearance.

Arterial blood gas sampling and interpretation

Specifications: An anatomical arm in lieu of a patient.

Before starting

- Introduce yourself to the patient.
- Explain the procedure and ensure that the patient consents to it.
- Check the case notes for anticoagulant treatment or platelet or clotting abnormalities.
- Note the patient's oxygen requirements and body temperature.
- Gather the required equipment in a tray.

The equipment

• Non-sterile gloves.	• Heparin 1000 U/ml (or a heparinised 2 ml syringe).
• Alcohol wipes.	• 23G (blue) needle (×2).
• Lignocaine 1%.	• Gauze.
• 2 ml syringe and cap for syringe.	• Sharps bin.

The procedure

- Wash and dry your hands or cleanse them with alcohol gel.
- Position the patient's arm so that the wrist is extended.
- Palpate the radial artery over the head of the radius and locate the site of maximum pulsation.
- Don the gloves.
- Cleanse the site with an alcohol wipe.
- Drape the area.
- Inject lignocaine intradermally around the chosen area, taking care not to puncture the vessel or mask its pulsation. (This step can be omitted depending on patient preference.)
- If you do not have a heparinised syringe, attach a 23G needle to the 2 ml syringe and draw up a little heparin into the syringe.
- Discard the needle into a sharps bin.
- Attach a second 23G needle to the syringe.
- Fix the chosen area between the index and middle fingers of your non-dominant hand.
- Warn the patient to expect a 'sharp scratch' or some other gross euphemism.
- Insert the needle at 30 degrees to the skin.
- Advance the needle a few millimetres in line with the direction of the artery until you obtain a flashback of bright red arterial blood into the syringe. Gentle aspiration from the syringe may in some cases be required.
- Allow the syringe to fill with 2 ml of arterial blood.
- Pick up a gauze with your non-dominant hand.
- Withdraw the needle and press firmly over the puncture site with the gauze. State that you would do this for 5 minutes, checking regularly for the formation of a haematoma.
- Discard the needle into a sharps bin.
- Expel any air bubbles from the syringe and cap it.
- State that you would immediately take the blood to a blood gas machine for analysis. At this point the examiner may hand you a print out from the machine.

After the procedure

- Ensure that the patient is comfortable.
- Interpret the print out, if any (see *Table 33*).
- Feedback to the patient/examiner.
- Ask the patient if he has any questions or concerns.
- Clear up.

Arterial blood gas interpretation (suggested approach for an OSCE station)

1. Assess PaO_2 (9.3–13.3 kPa, higher readings may indicate that the patient is receiving oxygen).
2. Assess pH

   ≤ 7.35 is acidosis.

   ≥ 7.45 is alkalosis.
3. Assess $PaCO_2$
   - If > 6.0 kPa there is either respiratory acidosis or respiratory compensation for metabolic alkalosis.
   - If < 4.7 kPa there is either respiratory alkalosis or respiratory compensation for metabolic acidosis.
4. Assess standardised HCO_3
   - If < 22 there is metabolic acidosis or renal compensation for respiratory alkalosis.
   - If > 28 there is a metabolic alkalosis or renal compensation for respiratory acidosis.
5. Combine information from 2, 3, and 4 above to determine the primary disturbance and whether there is any renal or respiratory compensation occurring (see *Table 33*).

Example

pH = 7.30

$PaO_2 = 6.8$

$PaCO_2 = 7.45$

$HCO_3 = 26.0$ mmol/l

This is uncompensated respiratory acidosis due to abruptly impaired ventilation, e.g. asthma attack.

Table 33. Arterial blood gas interpretation

	pH	$PaCO_2$	HCO_3
Respiratory acidosis	↓	↑	→, ↑*
Respiratory alkalosis	↑	↓	→, ↓*
Metabolic acidosis	↓	→, ↓**	↓
Metabolic alkalosis	↑	→, ↑**	↑
Mixed acidosis	↓	↑	↓
Mixed alkalosis	↑	↓	↑

* Renal compensation occurring.

** Respiratory compensation occurring.

Examiner's questions

Disorders of acid–base balance

Respiratory acidosis
- Results from alveolar hypoventilation.
- Common causes include airway obstruction, respiratory disease, impaired lung motion, neuromuscular disease, central nervous system depression, and obesity (Pickwickian syndrome).
- Symptoms are often those of the underlying cause, and in severe cases 'CO_2 narcosis' may supervene. Respiratory acidosis does not have a marked effect on serum electrolytes.
- Management involves oxygen therapy, but particular care must be taken in patients with COPD. Where possible, treat the cause.

Respiratory alkalosis
- Results from alveolar hyperventilation.
- Common causes include anxiety, pyrexia, CNS causes such as stroke and subarachnoid haemorrhage, liver failure, drugs such as salicylates and nicotine, high altitude, and mechanical ventilation.
- There may be signs and symptoms of hypocalcaemia (including positive Trousseau and Chvostek signs) without a fall in total serum calcium levels (due to increased binding of calcium).
- Management involves treating the cause.

Metabolic acidosis
- Results from increased production of hydrogen ions, or the inability to form bicarbonate in the kidney.
- Causes are various: some increase the anion gap and others do not. The anion gap (normal range 10–18 mmol/l) is a measure of organic acids and is given by $([Na^+]) - ([Cl-] + [HCO_3^-])$
- Causes that increase the anion gap include renal failure, massive rhabdomyolysis, diabetic ketoacidosis, lactic acidosis, and intoxication with ethanol or methanol.
- Causes that do not increase the anion gap include chronic diarrhoea and renal tubular acidosis.
- Symptoms are various and non-specific. In extreme cases there may be cardiac arrhythmias, and coma and seizures.
- Depending on severity, management may involve IV bicarbonate or dialysis.

Metabolic alkalosis
- Results from decreased hydrogen ion concentration or increased bicarbonate concentration.
- Principal causes include vomiting, diuretic treatment, hypokalaemia (due to intracellular shift of hydrogen ions), hyperaldosteronism, base ingestion, and over-compensation of respiratory acidosis.
- Symptoms include symptoms of hypocalcaemia (due to increased binding of calcium), symptoms of hypokalaemia (due to intracellular shift of potassium), hypoventilation, arrhythmias, and seizures.
- Metabolic alkalosis involving the loss of chloride ions is termed chloride responsive, because it typically corrects with IV administration of normal saline, whereas chloride-unresponsive metabolic alkalosis does not and typically involves severe hypokalaemia or mineralocorticoid excess.
- Treat the cause. Correct hypovolaemia and hypokalaemia. In severe cases, consider dialysis.

Station 102

ECG recording and interpretation

Before starting

- Introduce yourself to the patient.
- Explain the procedure to him, specifying that it is not painful, and ask him for his consent to carry it out.
- Position him so that he is lying on a couch.
- Ask him to expose his upper body and ankles.

The equipment

- A 12-lead ECG machine.
- Electrode sticky pads.

The procedure

- Indicate that you may need to shave the patient's chest to apply the electrode pads.
- Attach the electrode pads as per the leads.
- Attach the limb leads, one on each limb. The longest leads attach to the legs, above the ankles, and the mid-length leads attach to the upper arms.

Table 34. Colour codes for ECG limb and chest leads	
Limb leads	
Red	Right arm
Yellow	Left arm
Green	Left leg
Black	Right leg
Chest leads	
Red	V1
Yellow	V2
Green	V3
Brown	V4
Black	V5
Violet	V6

- Place the chest leads (the shortest leads) such that:
    - V1 is in the fourth intercostal space at the right sternal margin
    - V2 is in the fourth intercostal space at the left sternal margin
    - V3 is midway between V2 and V4
    - V4 is in the fifth intercostal space in the left mid-clavicular line
    - V5 is at the same horizontal level as V4, but in the anterior axillary line
    - V6 is at the same horizontal level as V4 and V5, but in the mid-axillary line
- Turn the ECG machine on and check calibration (1 mV = 1 cm in height) and paper speed (25 mm/s).

- Ensure that the patient is relaxed and comfortable and press on 'Analyse ECG' or a similar button.

Figure 82. Lead placement.

After recording the ECG

- Analyse the ECG for any life-threatening abnormalities.
- Remove the leads.
- Discard the electrode pads.
- Ensure that the patient is comfortable.
- Thank the patient.

Figure 83. Normal ECG.

ECG interpretation in 10 steps (suggested approach for an OSCE station)

Figure 84. The basic ECG complex.

1. Check labelling (name, date, calibration, paper speed, etc.) and eyeball the ECG.
2. Rate: divide 300 by the number of large squares between consecutive R waves.
3. Rhythm: ensure that each P wave is followed by a QRS complex. Use a pen and card to determine whether the rhythm is regular or irregular.
4. Axis:
   - normal axis: the QRS complexes are predominantly positive in both leads I and II
   - left axis deviation: the QRS complex is predominantly positive in lead I but is predominantly negative in lead II
   - right axis deviation: the QRS complexes are predominantly negative in both leads I and II
5. P waves: normal is less than 2.5 mm in height and 0.11 s in width in lead II.
6. PR interval: normal is 0.12–0.20 s or 3–5 small squares in duration.
7. QRS complex:
   - normal is < 0.12 s or 3 small squares in duration
   - the sum of the S wave in V2 and an R wave in V5 or V6 should not be greater than 35 mm
   - Q waves should not be deeper than one small square or 25% of the following R wave
8. ST segment: the ST segment should not be elevated or depressed.
9. T waves: T waves should not be tall, flattened, or inverted. T wave inversion in leads I, II, and V4–6 is always abnormal.
10. QT interval: normal is less than 400 ms or 2 large squares or half the R–R interval.

ECG interpretation in 10 easy steps – in more detail

1. Check **labelling** (name, date, indication, calibration 1 cm/mV, paper speed 25 mm/s).
2. **Rate:** either divide 300 by the number of large squares between consecutive R waves (1 large square = 0.2 s, 1 small square = 0.04 s) *or* count the number of R waves in the rhythm strip and multiply by 6 (as the rhythm strip is 10 s long).
   Sinus bradycardia (<~50 bpm and regular): athletes, hypothermia, hypothyroidism, intracranial hypertension, obstructive jaundice, SA node disease or ischaemia, beta blockade.
   Sinus tachycardia (>~90 bpm and regular): exercise, pain, fever, hypovolaemia, anaemia, pregnancy, thyroxicosis, vasodilators, vagolytics such as atropine.
3. **Rhythm:** ensure that each P wave is followed by a QRS complex. Use a pen and card to determine whether rhythm is regular or irregular. *Sinus arrhythmia* describes an increase in heart rate upon inspiration.
4. **Axis**
   a. *Normal axis*: the QRS complexes are predominantly positive in both leads I and II.
   b. *Left axis deviation*: the QRS complex is predominantly positive in lead I but is predominantly negative in leads II and III. Left axis deviation may indicate left anterior fascicular block and a number of other conditions, but not usually left ventricular hypertrophy.
   c. *Right axis deviation*: the QRS complexes are predominantly negative in both leads I and II. Right axis deviation may indicate right ventricular hypertrophy due to pulmonary conditions or congenital heart disease.

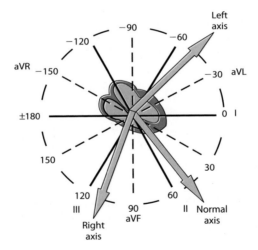

Explanation: normally the depolarising wave spreads towards leads I, II, and III and is therefore associated with a predominantly upward QRS deflection in all these leads, but greatest in lead II.

- In right axis deviation, the axis swings to the right so that the QRS deflection in lead I becomes negative and the deflection in lead III becomes most positive.
- In left axis deviation, the axis swings to the left, so that the deflection in lead III becomes negative. Left axis deviation is not significant until the deflection is also negative in lead II.

5. **P waves:** normal is less than 2.5 mm in height and 0.11 s in width *in lead II*. An inverted P wave in V1 is likely to indicate an incorrect recording. A tall P wave (P pulmonale) is due to right atrial enlargement and is seen most commonly in lung disease but also in tricuspid valve stenosis. A broad, bifid P wave (P mitrale) is due to left atrial enlargement and is seen most commonly in mitral stenosis.

6. **PR interval**: normal is 0.12–0.20 s (3–5 small squares) in duration. Prolonged in heart block, shortened in conditions involving an abnormality on the fibrous insulating ring such that signals get past the AV node more quickly, e.g. Wolff–Parkinson–White syndrome.

AV node blocks

- First degree block: atrial conduction is delayed such that the PR interval is consistently prolonged. This may be a sign of coronary artery disease, acute rheumatic carditis, digitalis toxicity, or electrolye disturbances.
- Second degree block: excitation completely fails to pass through the AV node. The causes of second degree heart block are the same as for first degree heartblock.
  - *Mobitz type I (Wenckebach phenomenon)*: there is progressive lengthening of the PR interval and then regular failure of conduction of an atrial beat, followed by a conducted beat with a short PR interval and then a repetition of this cycle.
  - *Mobitz type II*: most beats are conducted with a constant PR interval but occasionally there is an atrial contraction without a subsequent ventricular contraction. May herald complete heart block.

  - *2:1 (or 3:1) conduction*: there are alternate conducted and non-conducted atrial beats, giving twice (or three times) as many P waves as QRS complexes. May herald complete heart block in patients with MI.

- Third degree (complete) block: atrial contraction is normal but no beats are conducted to the ventricles. A ventricular escape rhythm takes hold, such that there is no relation between P and QRS. May occur after an MI (usually transient) or due to fibrosis around the bundle of His.

[Note] Heart block that is Mobitz type II or above requires pacing and is symptomatic (hypotension, dizziness, collapse). The choice between a temporary or permanent pacemaker depends on whether the underlying cause is transient or permanent.

SA node blocks can also occur but they are uncommon and usually asymptomatic (due to the establishment of a ventricular escape rhythm). SA node block is not to be confused with SA node *suppression*, which occurs when an arrhythmia prevents the SA node from generating an impulse.

7. **QRS complex:**
   a. Normal is <0.12 s or 3 small squares in duration. A broad QRS results either from depolarisation by a focus in the ventricular muscle or from a bundle branch block (BBB).
      i.   Right BBB: can be normal, or may be caused by IHD, PE, or ASD.
      ii. Left BBB: LBBB invariably reflects underlying heart disease, but its presence precludes further interpretation of the ECG.

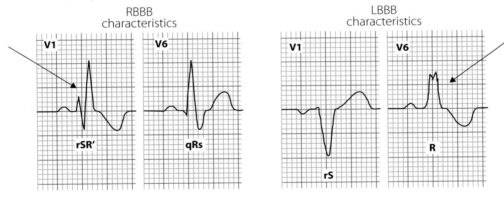

   b. The sum of the S wave in V2 and an R wave in V5 or V6 should not be greater than 35 mm. If it is, this indicates ventricular hypertrophy.
   c. Q waves should not be deeper than one small square or 25% of the following R wave. If they are, this indicates an old MI.

8. **ST segment**: the ST segment should not be elevated or depressed. Elevation of >1 mm indicates full thickness infarction of the myocardium.

    Depression of >0.5 mm indicates ischaemia, e.g. angina. In the presence of raised cardiac enzymes (e.g. troponin I) ST depression is indicative of MI (termed non-ST elevation MI). Saddle elevation in all the leads indicates pericarditis.
9. **T waves**: T waves should not be tall, flattened, or inverted. Tall, tented T waves indicate hyperkalaemia, flattened T waves indicate hypokalaemia. T wave inversion in leads I, II, and V4–6 is always abnormal, and indicates subendocardial (partial thickness) infarction, i.e. non-ST elevation MI, angina, or digoxin administration.
10. **QT interval**: normal is less than 400 ms (2 large squares) or half the R–R interval. Prolongation is usually secondary to drugs, e.g. antipsychotics, toxins, and electrolyte disturbances, and predisposes to potentially dangerous ventricular arrhythmias.

Abnormal rhythms

Supraventricular tachyarrhythmias (SVTs)

In SVTs the depolarisation spreads to the ventricles in the normal way via the His bundle so the QRS complex is normal and the same whether depolarisation was triggered by the SA node, the atrial muscle, or the junctional region.

Atrial extrasystoles

This example of atrial extrasystoles can be described as non-compensated atrial quadrigeminy: 'quadrigeminy' because there is one extrasystole after every three normal beats; 'non-compensated' because there is no compensatory pause after the extrasystole. Atrial extrasystoles are common in healthy people with normal hearts, and also occur in certain conditions such as cardiac failure and mitral valve disease.

Atrial tachycardia

In atrial tachycardia, there is a heart rate of about 150 with P waves superimposed on preceding T waves. Atrial tachycardia typically arises from an ectopic source in the atrial muscle and is often paroxysmal in nature. Although it is sometimes seen in patients with diseased hearts, it is nearly always benign.

Atrial flutter

In atrial flutter, the atrial rate is commonly 300 bpm and there is usually a 2:1 block, resulting in a ventricular rate of **150 bpm**. Can occur spontaneously in people with normal hearts, but most often occurs in people with cardiovascular disease. Frequently degenerates into AF.

Atrial flutter with *variable* (2:1 and 3:1) block. Fast P waves produce a 'saw-tooth' appearance.

Atrial fibrillation (AF)

AF is associated with any disease affecting the heart. There is an 'irregularly irregular' ventricular rate with no true P waves but baseline irregularities representing atrial activation.

AV nodal re-entrant tachycardia (AV 'junctional' tachycardia)

A re-entrant circuit is set up in the atria, causing the ventricles to depolarise at fast rates of up to 200 bpm. P waves are often absent, hidden in the QRS.

AV re-entrant tachycardia, via an accessory pathway e.g. Wolff–Parkinson–White syndrome

In WPW syndrome, some of the atrial depolarisation passes quickly to the ventricle before it gets through the AV node. The early depolarisation of the ventricle leads to a shortened PR interval and a slurred start to the QRS wave (delta wave).

Ventricular tachyarrhythmias

Ventricular extrasystole (VE)

Ventricular extrasystoles arise from an ectopic focus leading to a broad and atypical QRS complex that is unrelated to a preceding P wave. If a VE occurs early in the T wave of a preceding beat it can induce ventricular fibrillation.

Ventricular trigeminy.

Parasystole refers to a lack of coupling between VEs and the sinus rhythm. This may result in a number of fusion beats, in which a VE merges into the sinus beat.

Ventricular tachycardia (VT)

Two ventricular extrasystoles are termed a couplet but three or more are termed VT. Sustained VT can degenerate into ventricular fibrillation and death. Note the obvious dissociation between atria and ventricles.

* Accelerated idioventricular rhythm can look like VT, but the rate is <120 and the condition is benign. For this reason, VT should not be diagnosed unless the heart rate is >120.

** VT can be very difficult to differentiate from SVT with a BBB (as the BBB produces a broad QRS complex).

Ventricular fibrillation (VF)

Ventricular fibrillation is a chaotic ventricular rhythm which rapidly results in death.

Ventricular flutter

Ventricular flutter is a relatively uncommon and short-lived sine-wave like rhythm that usually degenerates into VF.

Bradycardias

Most abnormal rhythms are tachycardias, but they can also be bradycardias. The heart rate is normally controlled the SA node. However, if the SA node fails to depolarise, the heart rate is taken over by a focus in the atrial muscle or in the region around the AV node (the junctional region) both of which have spontaneous depolarisation frequencies of about 50 per min. If these also fail, or if the His bundle is blocked, the heart rate is taken over by a ventricular rhythm of about 30 per min. These slow, protective rhythms are collectively referred to as 'escape rhythms'. It is important to recognise them as such, because trying to suppress them can have dire consequences. The trace below shows a junctional escape rhythm:

ECG patterns

Myocardial infarction (MI)

In the 'hyperacute' phase, there are tall R waves and ST elevation which is sloped upwards and which often merges into tall, broad T waves. In established MI, there are prominent Q waves, elevated ST segments, and inverted 'arrowhead' T waves.

 In posterior MI, posterior wall changes are mirrored in the leads opposite the lesion, i.e. V1 and V2, leading to a tall R, ST depression, and upright 'arrowhead' T waves. Note that there may be no ECG changes in MI, so don't rely solely on the ECG!

Angina

ST segment depression of 1 mm or greater (Sheffield criteria) or ST elevation in Prinzmetal's angina.

Myocarditis

Tachycardia, atrial and ventricular extrasystoles, first degree and LAHB (left anterior hemi-block) heart blocks, ST changes.

Pericarditis

Sinus tachycardia, widespread 'saddle' elevation of the ST segment, T wave abnormalities.

Pericardial effusion

Diminished amplitude of ECG deflections and possibly also T wave inversion and electrical alternans (alternating QRS amplitude = tall one beat, short the next, and so on).

Pulmonary thromboembolism

Sinus tachycardia. Other ECG abnormalities are uncommon and the classical $S_IQ_{III}T_{III}$ syndrome only occurs in under 10% (prominent S in lead I, Q and inverted T in lead III). There may also be right atrial enlargement, atrial tachyarrhythmias, right ventricular hypertrophy or ischaemia, and RBBB.

Hyperkalaemia

Initially, tall tented T waves, then disappearance of P waves and, finally, broadened and distorted QRS complexes leading to ventricular arrhythmia or cardiac standstill.

Hypokalaemia

Flattened T waves and more prominent U waves which may be falsely interpreted as QT prolongation. There may also be first or second degree AV heart block.

Hypothermia

Sinus bradycardia, prominent 'J' wave, QRS and QT prolongation, leading to blocks, ventricular extrasystoles and, finally, VF.

> ⚠ *Try to familiarise yourself with different patterns of ECG, e.g. left ventricular hypertrophy, ischaemic heart disease, acute myocardial infarct, atrial fibrillation, heart block, pulmonary embolus. Study ECG libraries such as the one that can be found at www.ecglibrary.com/ecghome.html.*

Chest X-ray interpretation

A systematic approach to interpreting X-rays not only fills out the time and impresses the examiner, but also minimises your chances of missing any abnormalities. Before saying anything, it is an excellent idea to spend one minute looking at the X-ray, rubbing your chin and organising your thoughts.

Figure 85. Normal chest X-ray.

1. The X-ray

- Name and age of the patient.
- Date of the X-ray.
- PA, AP, or lateral?
- Erect or supine?
- Rotation – if there is no rotation, the distances from the vertebral spines to the medial ends of the clavicles should be equal.
- Penetration – if penetration is normal, the upper half of the thoracic spine should be discernible.

> **Erect or supine?**
>
> An X-ray can be confirmed as having been taken in the erect position if the gastric air bubble is found lying under the left hemidiaphragm.
>
> AP films are almost invariably taken supine, and this has major implications for interpretation. A supine film differs from an erect film in that:
>
> - there is an enlarged heart size
> - the diaphragm is higher, resulting in an apparent decrease in lung volume
> - pleural fluid levels lie vertically, resulting in an opacification of the lung field
> - any prominence of upper zone vessels does not suggest left heart failure

2. Interventions

Make a note of any chest drains, ECG pads, etc., that may be visible on the X-ray.

3. The skeleton

Inspect the ribs, the shoulder girdles, and the spine.

4. The soft tissues

Inspect the breasts, the chest wall, and the soft tissues of the neck. Look for any distortion, and for any opacities and translucencies.

5. The lungs and hila

The lungs: check the lung volumes, then carefully inspect the lung fields for any opacity or radiolucency.

The hila: inspect the hila, the densities created by the pulmonary arteries and the superior pulmonary veins of either lung for any abnormal opacities. Check their positions: the left hilum should be 2–3 cm higher than its right counterpart.

6. The pleura

Systematically check *all* lung margins, looking for pleural opacity, pleural displacement, and loss of clarity of the pleural edge (the so-called *silhouette sign*).

7. The diaphragm

Inspect the diaphragm and the area underneath it. The right hemidiaphragm should be at least 3 cm higher than the left.

8. The mediastinum and heart

First look for any mediastinal shift. Then calculate the cardiothoracic ratio (CTR) by dividing the maximal diameter of the heart by the maximal diameter of the chest. In a PA film the CTR should be 0.5 or less. Inspect the trachea and right and left main bronchi. Then inspect the aortic arch, the pulmonary artery, and the heart. Are there any abnormal opacities (masses) or radiolucencies (pneumomediastinum)?

9. Summarise your findings

Most common conditions likely to appear in a chest X-ray interpretation station	
Pneumonia	Pneumothorax
Pleural effusion	Lung cancer
Pulmonary oedema	Tuberculosis
Emphysema	Heart failure
Fibrosis	Rib fractures

 Learn their signs.

Abdominal X-ray interpretation

A systematic approach to interpreting X-rays not only fills out time and impresses the examiner, but also minimises your chances of missing any abnormalities. Before saying anything, it is an excellent idea to spend one minute looking at the X-ray and organising your thoughts.

Figure 86. Normal adult supine PA abdominal X-ray.

1. The X-ray

- Name, age, and sex of the patient.
- Date of the X-ray.
- Confirm size of area covered.
- PA or AP? (They are usually PA.)
- Supine (usual), erect, or lateral decubitus? (Look at gastric air bubble and fluid levels.)
- Penetration (lumbar vertebrae should be visible).

2. Interventions or artefacts

- Make a note of any clearly visible interventions or artefacts (*Table 35*).

Table 35. Abdominal X-ray: interventions and artefacts	
Interventions	Surgical clips, retained surgical instruments or swabs, nasogastric tube, CVP line, intrauterine contraceptive device, renal or biliary stents, endoluminal aortic stent, inferior vena caval filter
Artefacts/other	Pyjama bottoms, coins in pockets, body piercings, bullets, drugs ('bodypackers'), even, unfortunately, small animals

3. Skeleton

Inspect the:

- lower rib cage
- lumbar vertebrae
- sacrum and sacroiliac joints
- pelvis
- hip joints and femora

4. Organs

Inspect the:

- liver
- spleen: usually not visualised
- kidneys: about three vertebrae in size, the left kidney is higher than the right
- bladder: not visualised if empty
- prostate: only visualised if calcified
- stomach
- small bowel
- large bowel

 Large bowel usually frames a central area containing small bowel loops, not all of which are likely to be visible on an X-ray. If need be, large bowel and small bowel can be distinguished by their different mucosal markings: large bowel has haustra that cross only part of the bowel wall whereas small bowel has valvulae that cross its full width.

5. Gas, fluid levels, and faecal matter

- Gas: depending on its amount and distribution, intraluminal gas may be normal, but intra-mural or extraluminal gas should be considered abnormal. The small bowel should not be greater than 3 cm in diameter, the colon 5 cm in diameter, and the caecum 9 cm in diameter. Look for gas under the diaphragm (pneumoperitoneum), even though this is best visualised on an erect chest X-ray.
- Fluid levels: a fluid level in the stomach and caecum is a normal finding, but multiple fluid levels in the colon should be considered abnormal.
- Faecal matter: the amount and distribution of faecal matter can be revealing of underlying pathology.

6. Abnormal calcification

- Calculi (kidneys, ureters, bladder, gall bladder, and biliary tree).
- Pancreas.
- Kidneys.
- Abdominal aorta and arteries.
- Costal cartilages, although note that calcification of the costal cartilages is a benign finding in the older age population.

7. Summarise your findings

Most common conditions likely to appear in an abdominal X-ray interpretation station
Faecal impaction or overload
Obstruction (mass, stricture, volvulus, intussusception)
Ileus
Perforation
Biliary, renal, ureteric, or bladder calculi
Appendicolith
Artefacts (see *Table 35*)

Learn their signs, especially the barn-door ones such as apple-core and bird's beak.

Ordering investigations

Request forms for laboratory investigations (biochemistry, haematology, blood grouping and transfusion, microbiology, cellular pathology, immunology) and radiological investigations differ considerably from one hospital trust to another, so try to familiarise yourself with your local ones. Once you have seen the forms, they are actually pretty self-explanatory. Note that in some hospitals, investigations are ordered on a computer screen and paper forms are only used as a back-up.

On most forms you typically need to provide details about the:

Patient

- Last and first names
- Sex (usually 'M' or 'F', but sometimes 'U' for 'unknown')
- Date of birth
- Hospital number and NHS number

Use the patient's full name, e.g. 'Dorothy', not 'Dot or 'Dottie'. It is usually possible to omit the patient's hospital number and NHS number, but this is not best practice.

Request

- The ward or department that the report needs to go to ('Location for report'). Sometimes you are also able to specify a ward or department for a second copy of the report to go to ('Copy report').
- The speciality on behalf of which you are ordering the investigation, e.g. A&E, surgery.
- The name of the patient's consultant. If this is unclear, you can normally write the name of the consultant on take or on call.
- The patient's category (e.g. NHS, private, trial).
- The requesting doctor's name and signature.
- The requesting doctor's bleep or telephone number.

Specimen

- The type of specimen, e.g. blood, urine, sputum, other.
- Date and time of collection.
- The (anatomical) site of collection.

Clinical details

- The patient's clinical details, e.g.
  - chest pain, SOB, ECG changes, ? MI
  - pyrexia of unknown origin, ? cause
  - acute psychosis, due to start antipsychotic medication
- If the investigations are urgent, you can write 'Urgent please'. If the investigations are really urgent, take the sample and request form to the laboratory and speak to the technician in person.

On radiology request forms, you generally need to provide more specific clinical details, and specify what questions the examination should answer. You also need to specify the patient's transport (e.g. walking, chair, stretcher, bed) and other (e.g. oxygen, drip, escort) needs, and fill in a short risk assessment that is often in the form of a tick box list of questions (e.g. pregnancy, breast-feeding, allergies – yes/no).

Investigations requested

This obviously depends on the clinical situation. Commonly ordered laboratory and radiological investigations include FBC, haematinics, group and save, U&Es, LFTs, TFTs, glucose, lipids, CRP, ESR, amylase, D-dimers, blood cultures, MC&S, CXR, and AXR.

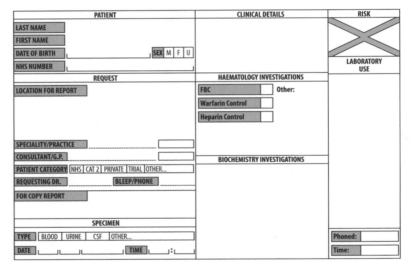

Figure 87. A typical request form for laboratory investigations. Note that, in this hospital, biochemistry and haematology investigations are requested on the same form.

After completing the request form

Before you take the specimen, confirm the patient's name and date of birth. For blood specimens, most hospitals use a purple specimen tube for haematology, a pink tube for group and save and cross-matching, a yellow tube for biochemistry (e.g. U&Es, LFTs, TFTs, CRP, lipids), a grey tube for glucose, a black tube for ESR, and a light blue tube for coagulation screen. Label the specimen tubes using a black ball-point pen, ensuring that the information on the label matches that on the request form. Place the labelled specimen tube into the bag on the reverse of the request form, remove the protective strip, and fold the flap onto the bag so as to seal it. Note that blood cultures require two 'blood bottles' with specific media for aerobic and anaerobic organisms.

VACUTAINER TUBE GUIDE – Draw tubes in the order given		
Haemoguard Stopper	**Tube Content**	**Determinations**
	SODIUM CITRATE 1:9	Coagulation Screen, Prothrombin Time (INR), APTT, Thrombophilia Screen, Lupus Anticoagulant Screen
	PLAIN (No Additive)	Anti-Cardiolipin antibodies
	SST	All Biochemistry Tests not mentioned elsewhere (1 Tube), Microbiology (1 Tube)
	HEPARIN	Chromosome Studies, Lead, Amino Acids, Troponin
	EDTA	FBC, Reticulocytes, Sickle Screen, Haemoglobinopathy Screen, G6PD, GF Test, Viscosity, Malarial Parasites, RBC Folate, ZPP, Marker Studies, Lead, Mercury Complement, Glycosylated Haemoglobin
	EDTA (cross match)	Blood Group, Save Serum, Crossmatch, Antibody Screening, Cord Blood Samples
	FLUORIDE/OXALATE	Glucose, Ethanol (Alcohol), Lactate
	SODIUM HEPARIN	Copper, Selenium, Zinc

Figure 88. Specimen tube guide. Note that the colours used may differ from one hospital trust to another.

Station 106

Drug and controlled drug prescription

Before prescribing a drug

- Look at the patient's medical notes. In particular, is there any hepatic or renal impairment/failure?
- Find out if he is on any other drugs, and consider possible interactions.
- Ask him if he has any allergies and document these in the medical notes.
- Explain to him the reason for recommending the drug, its likely beneficial effects, and its common or dangerous side-effects.

Prescribing a drug

- Write legibly and in black ink.
- Avoid all abbreviations other than those that are in common usage (see *Table 36*).
- Use generic names (unless a particular drug preparation is required).

Table 36. Latin abbreviations commonly used in prescribing drugs		
Abbreviation	**Latin**	**English**
OD	*omni die*	once a day
BD	*bis in die*	twice a day
TDS	*ter die sumendus*	three times a day
QDS	*quarter die sumendus*	four times a day
QQH	*quarta quaque horae*	every four hours
AC	*ante cibum*	before food
PC	*post cibum*	after food
OM	*omni mane*	every morning
ON	*omni nocte*	every night
PRN	*pro re nata*	as required
Stat.	*statim*	at once

Include:

- the date
- the full name, address, and date of birth of the patient
- the age of the patient if he is a child under the age of 12
- the generic name and formulation of the drug – prefer generic names unless a particular preparation is required
- the dose and frequency – avoid decimal points, e.g. 500 mg and not 0.5 g, and superfluous zeros, e.g. 4 mg and not 4.0 mg; if prescribing in micrograms, spell out 'micrograms' in full
- the minimum dose interval for PRN or 'as required' drugs only, e.g. cyclizine 5 mg 8 hourly
- the quantity to be supplied
- the signature of a registered medical practitioner – any alterations or mistakes should also be signed (or at least initialled)

Prescribing and administrative skills

Prescribing a controlled drug

In your own handwriting, include:

- the date
- the full name, address, and date of birth of the patient
- the generic name of the drug
- the formulation and strength of the preparation
- the required dose of the drug, frequency, and number of days it is to be taken
- the total amount of the preparation, or the total number of dose units in both words *and* figures
- your signature and address

December 12, 2007.

Mr John Adam Smith
42 West Register Street
London XXXX XXX

Date of birth: 01/09/1972

Methadone 10mg tablets   SPECIMEN
10mg TDS for 7 days
210mg, two hundred and ten milligrams in total.

Signed: Dr Peter Brown
The Best Hospital
London XXXX XXX

Prescribing on a hospital drug chart

- Hospital drug charts vary slightly from one hospital to another, so be familiar with your local ones. Most drug charts have four main sections, for regular drugs, PRN drugs, 'once-only' drugs, and fluids.
- Always write in black ink and in block capitals.
- Write at least the patient's name, date of birth, and any allergies/adverse reactions on every page of the drug chart.
- If prescribing a set course of medication, e.g. a 7-day course of antibiotics, cross off subsequent days so as to 'gate' the prescription.
- Sign and date every prescription. *If re-writing a drug chart, the date is not the date today, but the date on which the drug was first prescribed.*
- Record any changes you have made in the patient's case notes.
- Fluids and drugs such as oxygen, insulin and anticoagulants are sometimes prescribed on separate documents, and it is important not to miss them out if they have become separated from the drug chart.

 Avoid prescribing drugs you are unfamiliar with, high risk drugs such as anticoagulants and sedatives, and parenteral drugs without first consulting the British National Formulary *and senior colleagues.*

Example for a regular drug

PRESCRIPTION		Patient's Own Medicine	Date → Time →	1/7/08	2/7/08	3/7/08	4/7/08	5/7/08	6/7/08	7/7/08	8/7/08							
Medicine (Approved Name) LANZOPRAZOLE		For use	**6**															
			(8)	AB	AB	AB	AB	AB	AB									
Dose 30 mg	Route ORAL	Quantity	**12**															
Notes	Start Date 1/7/08	Date	**14**															
			18															
Prescriber – sign + print A Doctor A DOCTOR		Pharmacy	**22**															

Example for a PRN drug

PRESCRIPTION		Patient's Own Medicine		AS REQUIRED THERAPY					
Medicine (Approved Name) PARACETAMOL		For use	Date						
			Time						
Dose + Frequency 1 g 4–6 hourly Max 4 g/24 hrs	Route PO/BR	Quantity	Dose/Route						
			Initials						
Notes FOR PAIN	Start Date 1/7/08	Date	Date						
			Time						
Prescriber – sign + print A Doctor A DOCTOR		Pharmacy	Dose/Route						
			Initials						

Example for a once-only drug

			ONCE ONLY					
Date	Time	Medicine (Approved Name)	Dose	Route	Prescriber – Sign + Print		Time Given	Given By
1/7/08	0800	CEFUROXIME	1.5 g	IV	A Doctor	A DOCTOR	0800	AB
1/7/08	0800	METRONIDAZOLE	500 mg	IV	A Doctor	A DOCTOR	0800	AB

Example for fluids

		INFUSION THERAPY						

Date	Infusion solution	Additives and dose	Volume	Rate	Route	Sign	Time Given	Given By
1/07/08	Normal saline	None	1 l	8°	IV	A Doctor	0800	AB
1/07/08	Normal saline	None	1 l	8°	IV	A Doctor		
1/07/08	5% Dextrose	20 mmol KCl	1 l	8°	IV	A Doctor		

After prescribing a drug

- If you haven't done so already, give the patient instructions for administration of the drug.
- Ask the patient is he has any questions or concerns.

Table 37. Some commonly prescribed drugs and their adult dosages

Name	Dose	Frequency	Route(s)
Analgesics			
Paracetamol	1 g	4–6 h, max 4 g / 24 h	PO/PR
Diclofenac	50 mg	TDS	PO/PR
Ibuprofen	400 mg	QDS	PO
Cocodamol 8/500 or 30/500	2 tabs	QDS	PO
Codeine phosphate	30–60 mg	4 h, max 240 mg / 24 h	PO/IM
Tramadol	50–100 mg	4 h	PO/IM/IV
Morphine	5–10 mg	4 h	PO/IM/SC
Antibiotics			
Trimethoprim	200 mg	BD	PO
Penicillin V	250–500 mg	QDS	PO
Penicillin G	300–600 mg	QDS	IV
Amoxycillin	250–500 mg	TDS	PO
Co-amoxiclav 250/125 or 500/125	1 tab	TDS	PO
Flucloxacillin	25–500 mg	QDS	PO
Cefuroxime	250–500 mg	BD	PO
Cefuroxime	750 mg–1.5 g	TDS	IV/IM
Ciprofloxacin	250–750 mg	BD	PO
Clarithromycin	250–500 mg	BD	PO
Erythromycin	250–500 mg	QDS	PO
Metronidazole	400 mg	TDS	PO

continued

Table 37.   Some commonly prescribed drugs and their adult dosages – continued

Name	Dose	Frequency	Route(s)
Anticoagulants			
Tinzaparin DVT prophylaxis	3500 U	OD	SC
Tinzaparin DVT/PE treatment	175 U/kg	OD	SC
Dalteparin DVT prophylaxis	2500–5000 U	OD	SC
Dalteparin DVT/PE treatment	200 U/kg	OD	SC
Warfarin	As per hospital protocol and INR monitoring		
Antiemetics			
Cyclizine	50 mg	TDS	PO/IM/IV
Metoclopramide	10 mg	TDS	PO/IM/IV
Antihistamines			
Desloratadine	5 mg	OD	PO
Cetirizine	5–10 mg	OD	PO
Hypnotics			
Temazepam	10–20 mg	ON	PO
Zopiclone	3.75–7.5 mg	ON	PO
Proton pump inhibitors and antacids			
Lansoprazole	15–30 mg	OD	PO
Omeprazole	20–40 mg	OD	PO
Gaviscon®	10–20 ml	TDS	PO
Triple therapy (7 days)			
Lanzoprazole	30 mg	BD	PO ⎫
Amoxicillin	1 g	BD	PO ⎬
Clarithromycin	500 mg	BD	PO ⎭
Laxatives			
Lactulose	15 mls	BD	PO
Senna	2 tabs	ON	PO
Glycerin suppository	1–2	PRN	PR
Phosphate enema	1	PRN	PR
Movicol	1–3 sachets/day	Divided doses	PO
Other drugs			
Aspirin prophylaxis	75 mg	OD	PO
Simvastatin	10–40 mg	ON	PO
Bendrofluazide	2.5 mg	OD	PO
Lisinopril	2.5–20 mg	OD	PO

Oxygen prescription

Table 38. Guide to oxygen masks		
Type of mask	**Oxygen concentration**	**Indications**
Low flow masks		
Deliver a variable concentration of oxygen		
Nasal cannula	24–44% depending on the flow rate*	Patients with mild hypoxia who are otherwise stable; long-term domiciliary treatment
Simple face mask	Up to 60% at 6–10 l/min	Acutely breathless patients
Partial rebreather mask	60–80% at 10 l/min	As above
Non-rebreather mask	Up to 95% at 15 l/min	As above
High flow (Venturi) masks		
Deliver a fixed concentration of oxygen	24–60% in steps depending on the valve used (see *Table 39*)	'Carbon dioxide retainers' in whom oxygen control is a requirement**

* For every litre of flow delivered up to 6 litres, the oxygen concentration increases by about 4%, e.g. at 4 l/min, oxygen concentration is 36%.

**Note that the commonest cause of a high $PaCO_2$ is not carbon dioxide retention but ventilatory failure, in which the patient requires a high concentration of oxygen.

Table 39. Venturi mask valves		
Valve colour	**Flow rate (l/min)**	**Oxygen delivered (%)**
Blue	2	24
White	4	28
Yellow	6	35
Red	8	40
Green	12	60

Before starting

- Introduce yourself to the patient.
- Explain the need for oxygen and ensure that the patient consents to being treated.
- Quickly observe the equipment around you. There should be a selection of oxygen masks and Venturi valves.

The procedure

- Determine the patient's oxygen saturation using a pulse oximeter, and comment upon it.
- Tell the examiner that you would like to take an arterial blood gas sample. At this point, the examiner is likely to provide you with an arterial blood gas reading.

- Interpret the arterial blood gas reading (see *Station 101*).
- Select the appropriate piece of equipment and assemble it by connecting one end of the tubing to the piece of equipment and the other end to the oxygen source.
- Adjust the oxygen flow rate as appropriate.
- Apply the equipment to the patient, ensuring a tight yet comfortable fit.
- Tell the examiner that you would like to take a second arterial blood gas sample after a certain period of time. If the examiner provides you with a second arterial blood gas reading, interpret it and make the appropriate changes (if any).

After the procedure

- Record the instructions and sign the prescription chart.
- Ask the patient if he has any questions or concerns.
- Thank the patient.

Death confirmation

Golden lads and girls all must,
As chimney-sweepers, come to dust.

Cymbeline: Act II, Scene 2.
Shakespeare

Specifications: A mannequin in lieu of a cadaver (!)

- Take a history from a nurse (or indicate that you would do so) and consider the need for resuscitation.
- Ask for the patient's notes.
- Confirm the patient's identity: check his name tag.
- Observe the patient's general appearance and note the absence of respiratory movements.
- Ascertain that the patient does not rouse to verbal or tactile stimuli, such as pressure on a nail-bed.
- Confirm that the pupils are fixed and dilated.
- Use an ophthalmoscope to examine the fundi for segmentation of the retinal columns ('rail-roading' or 'palisading').
- Feel for the carotid pulses *on both sides*.
- Feel for the radial pulses.
- Feel for the femoral pulses.
- Auscultate over the precordium. Indicate that you would listen for one minute. Note whether the patient has a pacemaker or not (you can always look at a recent chest X-ray if you are not sure).
- Auscultate over the lungs. Indicate that you would listen for 3 minutes.
- Wash your hands.

 If any of your findings are non-corroboratory, you must consider the need for resuscitation.

- Make an entry in the patient's notes. Remember to include the time and date of death, and your examination findings.
- Indicate that you would:
  - consider the need for a post-mortem (see *Station 109: Death certificate completion*)
  - complete a death certificate (see *Station 109*)
  - inform the patient's GP and next of kin of the patient's death

Death certificate completion

 Legally, you can only fill in the death certificate if you have seen the patient in his last 14 days. Once the certificate is completed, it should be taken to the Registrar of Births and Deaths, usually by the patient's next of kin.

Before starting

You should understand the patient's history and the circumstances surrounding his death. You should have seen the patient's cadaver to confirm his death (or had the cadaver seen by a medically qualified colleague), noted if he had a pacemaker or radioactive implant, phoned his GP, and considered the need for a post-mortem examination (see *Table 40*).

Filling in the death certificate

In black ink, and as clearly and precisely as possible:

- Fill in the patient's:
    - name
    - date of death
    - age
    - place of death
- Fill in the date on which you last saw the patient alive.
- Circle one of the following statements:
    1. the certified cause of death takes account of information obtained from post-mortem
    2. information from post-mortem may be available later
    3. post-mortem not being held
    4. I have reported this death to the Coroner for further action
- Circle one of the following statements:
    a) seen after death by me
    b) seen after death by another medical practitioner but not by me
    c) not seen after death by a medical practitioner
- Fill in the cause of death: the disease that led directly to the patient's death is entered in Section I (a). The diseases that led to the disease entered in Section I (a) are entered in Sections I (b) and I (c).
- Fill in other significant diseases contributing to the death but not related to the disease having caused it in Section II.
- Tick the box if the death is related to employment.
- Sign the death certificate, fill in the date of issue, and print your name and medical qualification(s).
- Fill in the name of the consultant responsible for the overall care of the patient.
- Fill in the Counterfoil: record the patient's details and circumstances of death.
- Fill in the Note to Informant, and give it to the next of kin.

Table 40. Some reasons for referral to the coroner

The cause of death is uncertain.

The cause of death is due to industrial disease.

The cause of death is suspicious.

The cause of death is accidental.

The cause of death is violent.

The death is related to surgery or anaesthesia.

A doctor has not attended in the 14 days prior to the patient's death.

Clinical Skills for OSCEs

COUNTERFOIL

For use of Medical Practitioner, who should complete in all cases.

Name of deceased

Date of death

Age

Place of death

Last seen alive by me

Post-mortem?*   1   2   3   4
Coroner

Whether seen   a   b   c
after death*

Cause of death:—

I
(a)
(b)
(c)

II

Employment?   ☐ *Please tick where applicable*

B. Further information offered?

Signature

Date

Ring appropriate digit(s) and letter.

Register to enter
No. of Death Entry

☐

BIRTHS AND DEATHS REGISTRATION ACT 1953
(Form prescribed by the Registration of Births and Deaths Regulations 1987)

MEDICAL CERTIFICATE OF CAUSE OF DEATH

For use only by a Registered Medical Practitioner WHO HAS BEEN IN ATTENDANCE during the deceased's last illness, and to be delivered by him forthwith to the Registrar of Births and Deaths.

Name of deceased

Date of death as stated to me   Age as stated to me.

Date of death.   day of

Place of death.   day of

Last seen alive by me.

1   The certified cause of death takes account of information
     obtained from post-mortem.
2   Information from post-mortem may be available later.
3   Post-mortem not being held.
4   I have reported this death to the Coroner for further action.
     [See overleaf]

{ a Seen after death by me.
  b Seen after death by another medical practitioner
     but not by me.
  c Not seen after death by a medical practitioner.

Please ring appropriate digit(s) and letter.

CAUSE OF DEATH

The condition thought to be the 'Underlying Cause of Death' should appear in the lowest completed line of Part I

		These particulars not to be entered in death register
		Approximate interval between onset and death

I(a) Disease or condition directly
      leading to death†

(b)   Other disease or condition, if any,
      leading to I(a).

(c)   Other disease or condition, if any,
      leading to I(b).

II   Other significant conditions
      CONTRIBUTING TO THE DEATH but
      not related to the disease or condition
      causing it.

SAMPLE

The death might have been due to or contributed to by the employment followed at some time by the deceased.   ☐ Please tick where applicable

†*This does not mean the mode of dying, such as heart failure, asphyxia, asthenia, etc: it means the disease, injury, or complication which caused death.*

I hereby certify that I was in medical
attendance during the above named
deceased's last illness, and that the
particulars and cause of death above
written are true to the best of my
knowledge and belief.

Signature   Qualifications as registered
                             by General Medical Council }

Residence   Date

For deaths in hospital: Please give the name of the consultant responsible for the above-named as a patient

---

(Form prescribed by the Registration of Births and Deaths Regulations 1987)

NOTICE TO INFORMANT

I hereby give notice that I have this day signed a medical certificate of cause of death of

Signature

Date.

This notice is to be delivered by the informant to the registrar of births and deaths for the sub-district in which the death occurred.

The certifying medical practitioner must give this notice to the person who is qualified and liable to act as informant for the registration of death (see list overleaf). Where the informant intends giving information for the registration outside of the area where the death occurred, this notice may be handed to the informant's agent.

DUTIES OF INFORMANT

Failure to deliver this notice to the registrar renders the informant liable to prosecution. The death cannot be registered until the medical certificate has reached the registrar.

When the death is registered the informant must be prepared to give to the registrar the following particulars relating to the deceased:

1. The date and place of death.
2. The full name and surname (and the maiden surname if the deceased was a woman who had married).
3. The date and place of birth.
4. The occupation (and if the deceased was a married woman or a widow the name and occupation of her husband).
5. The usual address.
6. Whether the deceased was in receipt of a pension or allowance from public funds.
7. If the deceased was married, the date of birth of the surviving widow or widower.

THE DECEASED'S MEDICAL CARD SHOULD BE DELIVERED TO THE REGISTRAR

Prescribing and administrative skills

Complete where applicable

A

I have reported this death to the Coroner for further action.

Initials of certifying medical practitioner. ....

The death should be referred to the coroner if:

- the cause of death is unknown
- the deceased was not seen by the certifying doctor *either* after death *or* within the 14 days before death
- the death was violent or unnatural or was suspicious
- the death may be due to an accident (whenever it occurred)
- the death may be due to self-neglect or neglect by others

B

I may be in a position later to give, on application by the Registrar General, additional information as to the cause of death for the purpose of more precise statistical classification.

Initials of certifying medical practitioner. ....

- the death may be due to an industrial disease or related to the deceased's employment
- the death may be due to an abortion
- the death occurred during an operation or before recovery from the effects of an anaesthetic
- the death may be a suicide
- the death occurred during or shortly after detention in police or prison custody

LIST OF SOME OF THE CATEGORIES OF DEATH WHICH MAY BE OF INDUSTRIAL ORIGIN

MALIGNANT DISEASES

		Causes include
(a)	Skin	– radiation and sunlight – pitch or tar – mineral oils
(b)	Nasal	– wood or leather work – nickel
(c)	Lung	– asbestos – chromates – nickel – radiation
(d)	Pleura and peritoneum	– asbestos
(e)	Urinary tract	– benzidine – dyestuff manufacture – rubber manufacture
(f)	Liver	– PVC manufacture
(g)	Bone	– radiation
(h)	Lymphatics and haematopoietic	– radiation – benzene

POISONING

(a)	Metals	e.g. arsenic, cadmium, lead
(b)	Chemicals	e.g. chlorine, benzene
(c)	Solvents	e.g. trichlorethylene

INFECTIOUS DISEASES

		Causes include
(a)	Anthrax	– imported bone, bonemeal hide or fur
(b)	Brucellosis	– farming or veterinary
(c)	Tuberculosis	– contact at work
(d)	Leptospirosis	– farming, sewer or under-ground workers
(e)	Tetanus	– farming or gardening
(f)	Rabies	– animal handling
(g)	Viral hepatitis	– contact at work

CHRONIC LUNG DISEASES

		Causes include
(a)	Occupational asthma	– sensitising agent at work
(b)	Allergic alveolitis	– farming
(c)	Pneumoconiosis	– mining and quarrying – potteries – asbestos
(d)	Chronic bronchitis and emphysema	– underground coal mining

NOTE:—The Practitioner, on signing the certificate, should complete, sign and date the Notice to the Informant, which should be detached and handed to the informant. Where the informant intends giving information for the registration outside of the area where the death occurred, the notice may be handed to the informant's agent. The Practitioner should then, without delay, deliver the certificate itself to the Registrar of Births and Deaths for the sub-district in which the death occurred. Envelopes for enclosing the certificates are supplied by the Registrar.

PERSONS QUALIFIED AND LIABLE TO ACT AS INFORMANTS

The following persons are designated by the Births and Deaths Registration Act 1953 as qualified to give information concerning a death, in order of preference they are:

DEATHS IN HOUSES AND PUBLIC INSTITUTIONS

(1) A relative of the deceased, present at the death.

(2) A relative of the deceased, in attendance during the last illness.

(3) A relative of the deceased, residing or being in the sub-district where the death occurred.

(4) A person present at the death.

(5) The occupier* if he knew of the happening of the death.

(6) Any inmate if he knew of the happening of the death.

(7) The person causing the disposal of the body.

DEATHS NOT IN HOUSES OR DEAD BODIES FOUND

(1) Any relative of the deceased having knowledge of any of the particulars required to be registered.

(2) Any person present at the death.

(3) Any person who found the body.

(4) Any person in charge of the body.

(5) The person causing the disposal of the body.

*"Occupier" in relation to a public institution includes the governor, keeper, master, matron, superintendent, or other chief resident officer.

Figure 89. Copy of death certificate.

Station 110

Explaining skills

These skills can be used to explain a common condition, to explain an investigation, or to explain a procedure or treatment. They can also be used in your private life, although it may then be unwise to draw a diagram or hand out a leaflet.

What to do

- Introduce yourself.
- Summarise the patient's presenting symptoms.
- Tell the patient what you are going to explain.
- Determine how much the patient already knows.
- Determine how much the patient would like to know.
- Elicit the patient's main concerns.
- Deliver the information.
    - for a medical disorder: aetiology, epidemiology, clinical features, investigations/treatment, prognosis
    - for a pharmacological treatment: name, mechanism of action, procedure involved (dose, route of administration, frequency, precautions), principal benefits, principal side-effects, principal contraindications, alternatives including no treatment
    - for an investigative procedure: purpose, description of the procedure, principal risks, alternatives including no investigation, preparation required, after the procedure, results
    - for a surgical procedure: purpose, description of the procedure, principal risks, alternatives including no surgery, preparation required, anaesthetic procedure, post-operative care (e.g. recovery room, oxygen, blood pressure monitoring, etc.), analgesia
- Summarise and check understanding.
- Encourage and address questions.

How to do it

- Be empathetic.
- Explore the patient's feelings.
- Give the most important information first.
- Be specific.
- Regularly check understanding.
- Pitch the explanation at the patient's level. Use simple language and short sentences. If using a medical or technical term, explain it in layman's terms.
- Use diagrams, if appropriate.
- Hand out a leaflet.
- Be honest. If you are unsure about something, say you will find out later and get back to the patient.

What not to do

- Hurry.
- Reassure too soon.
- Be patronising.
- Give too much information.
- Use medical jargon.
- Confabulate (make things up).

"Really, now you ask me," said Alice, very much confused, "I don't think –"
"Then you shouldn't talk," said the Hatter.

Alice's Adventures in Wonderland: A Mad Tea-Party
Lewis Carroll

Some of the medical disorders, pharmacological treatments, investigative procedures, and surgical procedures that you may be asked to explain in an OSCE are listed below.
Information can be obtained from websites such as:
www.patient.co.uk
www.besttreatments.co.uk
www.kch.nhs.uk/patients/general-information/leaflets/

Medical disorders

- Asthma
- Diabetes
- Hypertension
- Angina
- Dementia
- Miscarriage
- Osteoarthritis/rheumatoid arthritis

Pharmacological treatments

- Statins
- Antibiotics
- Asthma inhalers
- Corticosteroids
- Insulin
- Antihypertensives
- Antidepressants
- Analgesics
- Glyceryl trinitrate
- Contraceptive pill (emergency pill, combined pill, progestogen-only preparations)
- Pessaries and suppositories
- Skin preparations, e.g. emollient, steroid cream, sunscreen

Investigative procedures

- Chest or abdominal X-ray
- CT scan
- MRI scan
- Ultrasound scan
- Echocardiography
- Flexible bronchoscopy
- Ventilation/perfusion scan
- Spirometry
- Oesophagogastroduodenoscopy (OGD)

- Barium swallow/meal/follow-through
- Barium enema
- Flexible sigmoidoscopy
- Colonoscopy
- Cystoscopy

Surgical procedures

- Angioplasty
- Laparoscopic cholecystectomy
- Endoscopic retrograde cholangiopancreatography (ERCP)
- Inguinal hernia repair
- Transurethral resection of the prostate (TURP)
- Hip/knee replacement
- Varicose vein stripping

Obtaining consent

Common questions

The purpose of gaining consent

Consent is needed on every occasion a doctor wishes to initiate an investigation or treatment or any other intervention, except in emergencies or where the law dictates otherwise (such as where compulsory treatment is authorised under the Mental Health Act).

How long is consent valid for?

Consent should be seen as a continuing process rather than a one-off decision. When there has been a significant period of time between the patient agreeing to a procedure and its start, consent should be reaffirmed.

Refusal of treatment

Competent adult patients are entitled to refuse treatment even when doing so may result in permanent physical injury or death. For example, a competent Jehovah's Witness can refuse a blood transfusion even if he will surely die as a result. An adult patient is competent if he can:

- Understand what the intervention is.
- Understand why the intervention is being proposed.
- Understand the alternatives to the intervention, including no intervention.
- Understand the principal benefits and risks of the intervention and of its alternatives.
- Understand the consequences of the intervention and of its alternatives.
- Retain the information for long enough to weigh it in the balance and reach a reasoned decision, whatever that decision may be. In some cases, the patient may not have the cognitive ability or emotional maturity to reach a reasoned decision, or may be unduly affected by mental illness.

Obtaining consent

 When seeking to obtain consent, it is important not to be seen to be rattling through a list of 'must dos', but trying to elicit the patient's ideas, concerns, and expectations, and tailoring your explanations accordingly.

- The type of information that should be provided to obtain consent includes:
  - what the intervention is (use diagrams if this is helpful)
  - why the intervention is being proposed
  - alternatives to the intervention, including no intervention
  - the principal benefits and risks of the intervention and of its alternatives
  - the consequences of the intervention and of its alternatives
- Ask the patient to summarise the above information, and be certain that he is competent to give consent.
- Remind the patient that he does not have to make an immediate decision and that he can change his decision at any time.

Station 112

Breaking bad news

What to do

- Introduce yourself.
- Look to comfort and privacy.
- Determine what the patient already knows.
- Determine what the patient would like to know.
- Warn the patient that bad news is coming.
- Break the bad news.
- Identify the patient's main concerns.
- Summarise and check understanding.
- Offer realistic hope.
- Arrange follow-up.
- Try to ensure there is someone with the patient when he leaves.

How to do it

- Be sensitive.
- Be empathetic.
- Maintain eye contact.
- Give information in small chunks.
- Repeat and clarify.
- Regularly check understanding.
- Give the patient time to respond. Do not be afraid of silence or of tears.
- Explore the patient's emotions.
- Use physical contact if this feels natural to you.
- Be honest. If you are unsure about something, say you will find out later and get back to the patient.

What not to do

- Hurry.
- Give all the information in one go, or give too much information.
- Use euphemisms or medical jargon.
- Lie or be economical with the truth.
- Be blunt. Words are like loaded pistols, as Jean-Paul Sartre once said.
- Prognosticate (*she's got six months, maybe seven*).

The angry patient or relative

I was angry with my friend:
I told my wrath, my wrath did end.
I was angry with my foe:
I told it not, my wrath did grow.

William Blake

The 'angry person' station can be rather unnerving, if only because medical students – and especially medical students in the earlier years of their training – are relatively sheltered from such persons.

The aim of the game is to diffuse the person's anger, *not* to ignore, placate or rationalise it. You should therefore try to be as empathetic and non-confrontational as possible.

What to do

- Introduce yourself.
- Acknowledge the person's anger.
- Try to find out the reason for his anger, e.g. frustration, fear, guilt.
- Validate his feelings.
- Let him vent his anger, or any feelings that led to his anger, e.g. frustration, fear, guilt.
- Offer to do something or for him to do something.

How to do it

- Sit at the same level as the person, not too close but not too far either.
- Make eye contact.
- Speak calmly and do not raise your voice.
- Avoid dismissive or threatening body language.
- Encourage the person to speak. Ask open rather than closed questions, and use verbal and non-verbal cues to show that you are listening.
- Empathise as much as you can.

What not to do

- Glare at the person.
- Confront him.
- Interrupt him.
- Patronise him.
- Get too close to or touch him.
- Block his exit route.
- Put the blame on others/seek to exonerate yourself.
- Make unreasonable promises.
- If the person is a patient's relative, be mindful of potential confidentiality issues.

The anxious or upset patient or relative

Are you upset little friend? Have you been lying awake worrying? Well, don't worry ... I'm here. The flood waters will recede, the famine will end, the sun will shine tomorrow, and I will always be here to take care of you.

Charlie Brown (to Snoopy)

What to do

- Look to comfort and privacy.
- Introduce yourself and try to establish rapport.
- Acknowledge the person's emotional state, e.g. *"You seem to be very upset."*
- Explore his feelings, e.g. *"What's making you so upset?"*
- Validate his feelings, e.g. *"I think that most people would feel that way in your situation."*
- Provide honest and accurate information about the situation.
- Offer to do something or for him to do something.
- Summarise and conclude.

How to do it

- Encourage him to speak, e.g. by asking open rather than closed questions and by prompting him on, e.g. *"Can you tell me more about that?"*
- Show that you are listening, e.g. by making appropriate eye contact, adjusting your body posture, and using appropriate verbal and non-verbal cues.
- Be empathetic.
- Use silence at appropriate times. If the person sheds tears, give him the time and space to do so and hand him a tissue.
- Use physical contact if this feels natural to you.
- Remain poised: speak calmly, use simple sentences, and pace the information that you give.
- Repeat and clarify the information that you give, and check understanding.
- Encourage questions.

What not to do

- Ask only closed questions.
- Interrupt or rush him.
- Do all the talking.
- Dismiss or trivialise his feelings.
- Reassure too soon.
- Offer inappropriate reassurance or false hope, e.g.
  - *"There's absolutely nothing to be afraid of, everything will be just fine."*
  - *"Sure she's dead, but you'll get over her much sooner than you think."*
  - *"I'm sure your father's in a better place now."*
- If the person is a patient's relative, be mindful of potential confidentiality issues.

Cross-cultural communication

You do not need to have a Masters in anthropology from the School of Oriental and African Studies to score highly in this station. All you need to do is use some basic communication strategies, as detailed here. It is also important that you are seen to respect the patient's beliefs and/or values.

- Introduce yourself to the patient, and ensure that he is comfortable.
- Ask the patient's name, age, and occupation.
- Determine the patient's reason for attending.
- Elicit the patient's:
  - **I**deas
  - **C**oncerns
  - **E**xpectations
    (**ICE**)
- Establish:
  - the patient's cultural or religious group
  - the implications that this has on his reason for attending
  - the patient's individual beliefs and values
- Check that you have understood the patient's problems.
- Explore possible solutions, and agree a mutually satisfactory course of action.
- Summarise the consultation.
- Check the patient's understanding.
- Thank the patient.

Communication skills

Station 116

Discharge planning and negotiation

Setting the scene

- Introduce yourself to the patient.
- Summarise the situation to him.
- Explore the impact that the illness/hospitalisation has had on him.
- Explore his current mood and disposition.

Going home and after

- Explain that you are considering for the patient to go home.
- Elicit and address any concerns that he may have about going home. Reassure him that transport can be organised, if need be.
- Explore his home situation and support system.
- Consider any extra help that can be offered to the patient, for example, social services, home help, *meals on wheels*, health visitor, district nurse, specialist nurses, palliative care team, dietician, occupational therapist, speech (language) therapist, physiotherapist, psychologist, continence advisor, self-help group, day centre.
- Discuss medication and compliance. Check that the patient doesn't have any concerns about taking his discharge medication and reassure him that the pharmacy can supply a Dossett box, if need be.
- Address risk factors. Suggest lifestyle changes that the patient may benefit from, such as stopping smoking, eating a balanced diet, taking regular exercise, etc.
- Offer the patient a follow-up appointment either at his GP surgery or in the Out-Patient Department.

Before finishing

- Summarise what has been said.
- Check the patient's understanding of what has been said.
- Ask the patient if he has any further questions or concerns.
- Thank the patient.